MAKING THE AMERICAN BODY

Making the American Body

The Remarkable Saga of the Men and Women Whose Feats, Feuds, and Passions Shaped Fitness History

JONATHAN BLACK

UNIVERSITY OF NEBRASKA PRESS | LINCOLN AND LONDON

∞

Library of Congress
Cataloging-in-Publication Data
Black, Jonathan, 1943–
Making the American body:
the remarkable saga of the men
and women whose feats, feuds,
and passions shaped fitness
history / Jonathan Black.
pages cm
Includes bibliographical
references and index.
ISBN 978-0-8032-4370-5
(cloth: alk. paper)
1. Physical fitness—United States—
History. 2. Health attitudes—United
States—History. I. Title.
GV510.U5B53 2013
613.7—dc23 2013008307

Set in Minion by Laura Wellington.
Designed by Nathan Putens.

For Adrian and Lucian

Contents

Preface

Fitness today is an all-consuming habit. Untold millions troop to health clubs or run on paths and tracks or work out at home on equipment peddled on late-night infomercials. Yoga is experiencing an unprecedented boom. There are Pilates studios and boot camps and Zumba parties. There are fitness facilities in every hotel, in corporate centers and tennis clubs, in spas and on cruise ships. Exercise touches every aspect of our culture, from books and magazines to television shows and high-end clothing boutiques. How we arrived at this state of heightened awareness is a story whose contours mirror much that happened in twentieth-century America, but it is also, on another level, the tale of individuals. Virtually no other habit or business has been so propelled, and for so long, by such a remarkable cast of characters.

As diverse as they were, all shared a singular passion — to improve on the human body. Some happened on their mission by chance. Many latched on to exercise to overcome an early life that was blighted by illness, deprivation, or low self-esteem. Not surprisingly, few believed in moderation and fewer still in humility. Proud of their new physicality, they were big on self-promotion. The early icons with bodybuilder roots were the most likely exhibitionists, but shifting notions of fitness did little to alter their profile; almost all were crusaders with outsized egos and a flair for showmanship, and their occasional clashes made for enduring feuds and high comedy.

Singly and together, they shaped the habit of exercise in America, but their influence extended beyond the treadmill and yoga mat. They impacted advertising and figured large in the early use of television. They helped spawn the videotape industry. At a time when the demographics of the country were shifting, from rural to urban, they offered hubs for immigrants and a source of identity and confidence. In the daily shuttle between home and office, they introduced a new "third place," the health club, a source of friendship and social interaction. The promise they offered, of personal transformation, touched a common feature of the American dream — that anyone, with will and determined effort, could be a success and live a happier, more fulfilling life.

It can be said that their feats and stories fit no single narrative, that the very notion of a history of fitness weaves a misleading theme. The early "muscle heads" had little in common with the millions of converts to jogging; the addicts of Spinning would never deign to sit in the adjacent yoga studio. But this segmentation overlooks the progression that defines how Americans look at their bodies and how they employ them to further a sense of accomplishment and well-being, because most everything chronicled here was built on something that came before. The very notion of "fitness" appeared late in the game, but its provenance dates back to muscular Christianity and the nutritional zealots of the nineteenth century; it developed in the showmanship of Mr. Olympia contests and the drive to do better in sports; it fed off a national slump in self-confidence and the need to look good in the aerobics studio; it was a natural outgrowth of the coupling of exercise and health.

The end result of this history, it is fair to argue, has failed to fulfill its promise. The country is in the midst of an obesity epidemic, diabetes is on the rise, and so is the incidence of heart attack and stroke. One might conclude that the heroes of this book are partly to blame — for their salesmanship and commercialism, for their occasional grandiosity and excesses. To do so, however, would be to overlook how far they have brought us. Their flaws and limitations need not detract from the vision and vitality that inspired so many. What they accomplished should set a standard for our own ambitions — and what still needs to be done.

Introduction | A Night to Remember

There was plenty of entertainment in New York City that warm night in October 1924. Up in Times Square, the Ziegfeld Follies were playing at the New Amsterdam, the marquee proclaiming, "A National Institution! Glorifying the American Girl!" Around the corner, Gloria Swanson was starring in the Broadway smash *The Impossible Mrs. Bellew*. Harold Lloyd was cracking them up in his latest five-reel comedy riot, *Grandma's Boy*. Marion Davis was in her "sixth capacity week" in *When Knighthood Was in Flower*.

But for fans of something different, for connoisseurs of male flesh and muscle, there was only one place to be that night—Madison Square Garden. This was the second Garden, the one designed by Stanford White, a huge, sprawling Moorish palace with a thirty-two-story minaret overlooking Madison Square at Twenty-Sixth Street. Atop the minaret an eighteen-foot bronze statue of a nude Diana had originally spun with the wind; deemed too erotic and possibly a danger to passersby below, it had been replaced with a much lighter, gilded hollow copy. The Garden's rooftop restaurant was the city's largest, as famous for its food as for the night when Henry K. Thaw shot White dead at his table because the architect had been having an affair with Thaw's wife, Evelyn Nesbit, much of it carried on in the apartment that White kept in the building, the site of the notorious red-velvet swing.

The Garden was the only place big enough to accommodate the likely crowds. Its main hall was enormous, the largest in the world, with seating capacity for eight thousand people and floor space for thousands more. In recent years, the Garden had played home to all manner of shows—rodeos and circuses and speed-walking races. It rarely made back its money, however, and entrepreneur Tex Rickard took over the arena to introduce the new sport of boxing. The night before, record-breaking numbers of fans witnessed a tough kid from Chicago, Charlie White, flatten the Canadian lightweight champ with a jackhammer left one minute into the second round.

There would be no fisticuffs tonight, but there would be plenty of macho display. Seventy-five men from around the world were here to show off their rippling abs and tree-trunk thighs. It was billed as "The World's Most Perfectly Developed Man" contest, and tickets were hard to come by.

The crowds had been lining up for hours. Policemen patrolled the lines brandishing night sticks. Brokers were waving tickets, yelling for more. Inside, in the basement dressing rooms, dozens of men methodically stripped off their clothes to begin their preshow ritual. Off came a shirt, the body turned sideways to the mirror, an arm cocked, the tight-roped bicep regarded with squinted satisfaction. Bodies hunched forward; shoulders leaped to life. A massive chest, a pulverizing clot of muscle, sprang into profile. Only the occasional grunt of confidence broke the tense silence.

Few noticed the dressing-room door crack open and the head of a man appear. The man was handsome, with a sharp aquiline nose, a high forehead, and piercing blue eyes. The narrow lips were fixed in their usual arrogant expression. He was dressed in a suit, though had he stripped off his clothes he would have appeared every bit as striking as the muscled Adonises in front of their mirrors. Short, a mere five-foot-two, he boasted an impressive physique, his powerful arms thickened by hundreds of morning push-ups, his stomach tightened by thousands of sit-ups. He lived by one credo, emblazoned under the banner of his best-selling magazine, *Physical Culture*: "Weakness Is a Crime. Don't Be a Criminal."

His name was Bernarr Macfadden.

He was, by most any account, the strangest man to leave his mark on the world of fitness—and one of the most influential. He educated the world about alternative medicine, proper nutrition, sex. He founded a utopian community and built luxury health sanatoriums. In years to come, he would create a hugely successful publishing empire with magazines such as *True Story* and *True Confessions*. He would persuade the nation's first lady to edit his magazine on babies and would declare himself a candidate for president.

Tonight he was trading on the title that had made him famous: the self-appointed "Father of Physical Culture." It was an unlikely crown for the man who had grown up weak and sickly in the Ozarks. An orphan, he had transformed himself through fanatic devotion to exercise and had become America's greatest promoter of health foods and clean living. He abstained from smoking, alcohol, and drugs. He campaigned against prudery and believed sex prevented baldness. He slept on his bedroom floor and walked six miles to work, barefoot. He shaped his body as he shaped his life – with a disregard for moderation. He borrowed what suited him. The term *physical culture* had been popularized by the world's greatest bodybuilder and dated back to the nineteenth century, its provenance owed to a rediscovery of the body and a rebellion against Victorian restraint. In the twentieth century, it gathered a new momentum in the military, in schools, even in churches, fusing exercise with health and even spirituality.

Macfadden was quick to capitalize on the new "Body Worship," as it had come to be called. At the time of the Madison Square Garden event, the country was still recovering from the carnage of World War I, and many had turned to the human body as one means to establish control over a more limited canvas. The advent of photography had further propelled display of the sculpted male form, and Macfadden made the most of this new interest by running provocative pictures in *Physical Culture*, a strategy that worked both for and against him. Advertisements for an earlier show, his "Mammoth Physical Culture Show – a Carnival of Beauty and Brawn," had caught the eye of antivice zealot Anthony Comstock, who had him arrested for passing around photos of women in swimsuits. Macfadden got a suspended sentence but ran afoul of the law again by running an explicit series of photos on the dangers of syphilis in *Physical Culture*. Only a reprieve from President Taft saved him from a two-year prison term.

For tonight's extravaganza, he was determined to cloak the near-naked men in respectability and had recruited a blue-ribbon panel of judges, which included doctors, scientists, and nutritionists. If all went as planned, the event would garner the kind of publicity that Macfadden craved – for himself, naturally, but also for the doctrine of physical culture. Looking around him, he was appalled at the wretched condition of so many men. Weak, out of shape, they stumbled through their lives ignorant of the body's potential. He, Bernarr Macfadden, had been put on the planet to restore the glow of good health and the miracles of a powerful body.

From his position at the door, he surveyed the muscles that coiled and bulged under dressing-room lights. It was a beautiful sight, the body's benediction to his tireless work and obvious genius. He had only one reservation: tonight's event was a charade. All these men with their glorious oiled bodies were wasting their time. The winner who would soon walk off with the title of "World's Most Perfectly Developed Man" was a foregone conclusion. Quietly, he shut the door and went to find him in another dressing room.

The man had come to Macfadden's attention one year ago, when the publisher was promoting a photo contest, the "World's Most Beautiful Man," in the pages of his magazine. The picture the man sent had impressed Macfadden, but so had many of the photos that poured in through the mail. It was a difficult decision, and three months passed before he had replied to the contestant, suggesting he come by Macfadden's office in midtown Manhattan for a personal inspection.

The man had arrived in a business suit. He had a handsome square face, his eyes bright but calm. If he was nervous, he did not show it. Macfadden, ever attuned to physical auras, sensed a reserve of strength. The hair was obviously healthy, important to Macfadden, who sported a spongy black pompadour, evidence of his prophylactic cure for baldness. Even seated in a chair, legs casually crossed, the man emanated something special. There was the obvious bulge of his shoulders where they strained the suit jacket. His grip had been sure, confident — not the kind of crude, bone-crushing shake meant to impress. Macfadden was pleased to learn the man shared many of his values; he neither drank nor smoked. He spoke English well, not a trace of an accent, though he had apparently come from some tiny town in southern Italy. Most surprising was the man's description of how he had attained the body concealed beneath his clothes. If he was to be believed, the man had developed himself without use of barbells or dumbbells. There had been no machines.

This impressed Macfadden. He had invented an exercise machine himself, but did not believe in gadgetry. The body God had crafted provided all the tools needed — so long as the blood remained pure. He offered the man a glass of carrot juice. There arrived the moment of truth.

"Alright," said Macfadden. "Let's have a look."

A few moments later the man stood before him, naked but for a pair of tight leopard underpants. Macfadden blinked in disbelief.

"You did this . . . without weights?"

"Yes, sir."

"But at a gym, yes?"

"No gym, sir. I developed myself at home."

The broad shoulders, muscled but not larded with flesh, tapered to a trim waist. The sculpted chest seemed almost unreal, as if expanded from within by a divine hand. The river of muscles from thigh to calf suggested thousands of squats, the kind Macfadden performed every morning.

"Could you . . ."

Obligingly, the man turned to profile and flexed his arm. Macfadden had never seen such biceps. The forearms . . . the tensed muscles that seemed to vibrate up and down his back . . . the casual strength that emanated from this man like . . . like a Greek god.

Macfadden told him to put his clothes back on. He only half-listened as the man described what had drawn him to bodybuilding . . . a childhood not unlike his own, growing up weak and spindly and bullied. His determination to change all that, the revelation he had at the Brooklyn Museum in front of a famous statue, his time at the sideshows at Coney Island, where he'd first heard of the Prussian strongman Eugen Sandow.

He went to his desk and took a checkbook out of a drawer. He wrote in the amount without hesitation, glancing up only once to make certain this marbled vision, this man he had only dreamed of, was not a mirage.

"Here's a thousand dollars," he said. "It's the prize. You win."

"Thank you, sir."

"And the name. I need to fill in the name. Again, it's . . ."

"Angelo Siciliano."

"I thought it was something different."

"That's the name I was born with. Now it's Charles Atlas."

Charles Atlas, he thought. It was a heavy burden to lift the weight of the world. But Bernarr Macfadden had a feeling, and he was never wrong.

MAKING THE AMERICAN BODY

CHAPTER 1

The Shape of History

All credit to the Greeks; muscular Christianity; pioneers on the Continent—and at Harvard; the zealots of nutrition

The ideal of the perfect body, no surprise, goes back to ancient Greece, as does the start of what we now call fitness. There is evidence that the Egyptians were big on acrobatics and related training as far back as 2100 BCE, and not long after the Chinese introduced Cong Fu, a means of promoting health through breathing and fluid body movements. But it is to Greece that we owe our image of the sculpted male form—largely because those forms survive in marble. It is to Greece that we owe the word *gymnasium*—from the Greek *gymnos*, meaning "naked," which was how the Greeks exercised.

The Greek gymnasium was about more than exercise. It promoted the ties between athletics, education, and health, and the great public gymnasiums of Athens were the favored open-air lecture halls of philosophers. When not absorbing the wisdom of Plato and Aristotle, Greeks came to indulge their love of sport and athletic contests, which culminated in the Olympics. Footraces of all types and lengths were a major Olympics attraction, though never the marathon. That race owes its provenance to Pheidippides, the Greek messenger who ran from Athens to Sparta to beg for help fighting the Persians, who had landed at Marathon, then ran back to Athens to proclaim victory—whereupon he collapsed and died.

Herodotus, it needs noting, was a reliable battlefield chronicler and makes no mention of Pheidippides, stressing instead the intervention of the god Pan. Quite possibly the Athenians chose to minimize their reliance on Sparta, whose citizens were deemed narrow-minded and boorish, interested in fitness only as it served their military. At age seven, Spartan males were whisked away to tough training schools and a lifetime of soldiering.

It was not just sport that powered the Athenian passion for exercise. Hippocrates was a big believer in proper nutrition and physical activity. "Walking is man's best medicine," he said. Millennia ahead of his time, he declared: "If we could give every individual the right amount of nourishment and exercise, not too little and not too much, we would have the safest way to health." Plato had much the same advice. "Lack of activity destroys the good condition of every human being, while movement and methodical physical exercise save and preserve it."

With the collapse of Greek civilization, the ideal of the body beautiful and the attendant need for exercise went into serious hibernation. The Roman motto of "a healthy mind in a healthy body"—*mens sana in corpore sano*—was espoused mostly in the service of warlike goals and the need to truck heavy weapons into brutal battle. The long sweep of the Middle Ages, however interesting for its religiosity, architecture, and feudal hierarchies, paid scant heed to developing the body. The challenges of survival in the face of famine, plagues, and a minor ice age were distraction enough. It was not until the Renaissance that attention returned to the naked human form, in large part thanks to the study of anatomy by Leonardo da Vinci and Michelangelo. Even then, the casual grace of a *David*, say, or the tensile muscularity of a *Moses* or *Medici*, was largely an abstract ideal to be admired—never an actual prototype for the common man. For that, one needs to leapfrog another few centuries, over the age of exploration and the Enlightenment, over the costumed indulgences of the French Empire, and on into the nineteenth century, when fascination with Greece again blossomed.

So-called Greek Revivalism started as an interest in architecture but boomed in 1807 with the display of the Elgin Marbles in London. As more Greek sculptural treasures were plundered, public fascination with Greece turned to classical education and its focus on physical training and athletic competition, and it was not long before schools were offering "Greek gymnastics." Heading up the most influential of these schools in Germany, Johann GutsMuths penned what is arguably the first bible of fitness, a seven-hundred-page tome entitled *Gymnastics for Youth; or, A Practical Guide to Healthful and Amusing Exercise for the Use of Schools.* With chapter titles such as "We Are Weak Because It Does Not Occur to Us to Be Strong," GutsMuths rooted his ideal in "the Greeks [who] were eminent for beauty and symmetry of form. Not only were they all exercised but those more especially which most required exercise. . . . Thus they grew to their natural proportions; thus the muscles welled up to a beautiful and manly firmness." To achieve that perfection, he detailed a lot of information about running, leaping, wrestling, and lifting.

The gospel was spread by another German, Friedrich Ludwig Jahn, a gymnastics instructor and rabid nationalist. Mortified by Napoleon's defeat of Prussia in 1806, as were most Germans, he campaigned for renewed strength and freedom, going so far as to live in a cave and sport a bearskin on the streets of Berlin. He eventually started a militaristic school that linked exercise and sport to German history and launched what was arguably the world's first gymnastic club, the Turn (often called Turnverein). Most remarkably, he filled it with equipment he invented that still defines the sport: the pommel horse, parallel and horizontal bars, and vaulting blocks, as well as dumbbells and Indian clubs. His fanatic anti-Semitism and hatred of the French, unfortunately, did not sit well with the more liberal German Confederation of Metternich, and the Turnvereins were soon closed and the apparatus dismantled. Jahn himself was imprisoned and barred from teaching or gymnastic work after his release in 1825. A more liberal atmosphere in the 1840s revived the Turnvereins, and by 1860 there were more than 150 around the globe.

France had its own celebrity entrepreneur, a man named Hippolyte Triat who opened a Paris gymnasium that presaged, both as a workout space and as a business, the upscale health clubs of the twentieth century. His biography would have been fantastic enough: an orphan, he was kidnapped at age six by Gypsies and forced to wear a dress while performing in a wire-walking act as "Young Isela." Released finally, he joined a Spaniard who had formed a weightlifting troupe with his sons and then—more good fortune!—rescued a rich lady on a runaway horse and was rewarded with tuition to an elite Jesuit college. A convert now to theatrical spectacle as well as deep-pocket sponsors, he stunned Paris with a vast vaulted hall and filled it with every conceivable apparatus—and many new ones he invented. Well-heeled spectators were encouraged to watch from side galleries as instructors led bare-chested men in synchronized routines to the beat of drums. All of high society made a pilgrimage to Triat's gymnasium, as did much of the royal court of the Second Empire, including the emperor, to whom Triat personally tended. The less privileged could buy shares and redeem them for memberships or to pay for private lessons. Triat's enterprise had a few problems—its expenses, the complexity of routines, Triat's radical politics that led him to join the Paris Commune. In its bloody aftermath, his gym was confiscated and Triat briefly imprisoned at Versailles. He died a forgotten man in despair and poverty, the genius of his foresight shelved for a good 150 years until the advent of mirrored studios in American health clubs and the boom in personal training and group exercise.

America, mid-nineteenth century, had picked up the exercise habit, thanks largely to European models. In 1848, riding the wave of German immigrants, the first Turn opened in the United States in Cincinnati, and St. Louis quickly followed. Czech immigrants started their own versions of the Turnverein called Sokols. Two athletic clubs, the Olympic Club of San Francisco and the New York Athletic Club, opened in 1860 and 1868, respectively.

The social aspect was key. As the Industrial Revolution picked up steam, Americans increasingly crowded into cities. By 1850 more than 40 percent of the population had moved off the land and into urban environments. For people used to the simple rigor of field work and farms, cities could be intimidating places: impersonal, confusing, even dangerous. With the 1848 revolutions in Europe, waves of immigrants packed into slums. The gymnasium offered a home to new arrivals, a place to get to know their neighbors and at the same time learn ways to combat the health and moral hazards of the scary city. For many, gyms and athletic clubs took the place of a church, especially with the spread of what became known as "muscular Christianity."

The term derived from the works of the popular English novelist Thomas Hughes, whose young fictional hero, Tom Brown, was renowned for his active life and exploits. "[It is] a good thing to have strong and well exercised bodies," wrote Hughes in *Tom Brown at Oxford*. "The least of the muscular Christians has hold of the old chivalrous and Christian belief that a man's body is given to him to be trained and brought into subjection, and then used for the protection of the weak [and] the advancement of all righteous causes." (Curiously, it was another book in Hughes's series that inspired the first modern-day Olympic Games. In *Tom Brown at Rugby*, the smallish boy goes off to boarding school at Rugby, where he participates in athletics, helping him thrash the school bully. The climax of the novel is a game—cricket. A Frenchman and rabid Anglophile, Pierre Fredy, was so taken with the story that he made a pilgrimage to Rugby and then devoted his life—and fortune—to restoring the Games, declaring, "For me, sport is a religion with church, dogma, ritual." Ascending to the title of the Baron de Coubertin, he played a key role in persuading the Greeks to hold the first modern Olympics in 1896—and convinced them to make Athens only the first stop in a quadrennial global road show.)

The words *muscular Christianity* first appeared in an 1857 *Saturday Review* critique of the book *Two Years Ago* by another English novelist, Charles Kingsley. Though he initially balked at the term, Kingsley soon became its most fervent popularizer, writing, "Games conduce not merely to physical but to moral health." His insistence that morality was a function of muscularity as well as piety—the best Christian, said Kingsley, was a physically fit Christian—reflected a founding principle of the Young Men's Christian Association. The first YMCA chapter in the United States, modeled after a London club, was started by an American seaman and missionary, Captain Thomas Sullivan, to provide a "home away from home" for young sailors on leave. It opened in Boston in 1851 and promoted evangelical Christianity, stressing the linked importance of mind, body, and spirit—symbolized in the distinctive YMCA triangle. That emblem was designed by a YMCA training instructor, Luther Gulick, the most prominent devotee of muscular Christianity, who contended, "Bodily vigor is a moral agent."

Sport and physical training, went the belief, rechanneled the energy that steered young men to slack behavior and crime. There was added urgency when Frederick Jackson Turner formally announced the "death of the frontier" in 1893. A fast-civilizing West deprived people of a natural outlet for aggression, particularly the swelling urban populations. The growth of organized sports in college added steam to the so-called Athletic Revival, as did new sports. Both volleyball and basketball were invented in the 1890s, the latter at the YMCA training facility at

Springfield College in Massachusetts. Calisthenics became popular, especially among women. The bicycle appeared in the late 1800s and soon became a craze. Though maligned by some for encouraging masturbation and sex, riding was hailed as a cure-all for everything from neurasthenia to consumption.

In the years following the Industrial Revolution, building a muscular body acquired a new appeal; as one social historian explained it, "Muscular posing's conflation with simply physical strength [was] a push against the prevailing experience of a machine age in which the body was in some ways less exalted as a productive resource." Any activity caught the public fancy. Among the more captivating trends was the habit of endurance walking, thanks largely to the exploits of Edward P. Weston. Tagged "Weston the Pedestrian," he turned his marathon hikes into crowd spectacles with the added interest of wagers and once walked from Portland, Maine, to Chicago to win a ten-thousand-dollar bet.

The body acquired a new reverence in the unlikely ivied halls at Harvard. There a slightly built fellow named George Windship entered medical school as the second smallest in his class of 1854. Presaging the legend of Charles Atlas, who had sand kicked in his face and swore revenge, Windship was humiliated when a classmate threw his books down a staircase. To right the wrong, and determined to avenge himself on the bully, he built himself into a rock-hard specimen by lifting weights and billed himself as the "Roxbury Hercules." He operated a large gymnasium in Boston where he also conducted his medical practice and sold apparatuses, including the "Windship Patent Graduating Dumb-Bell."

Windship's celebrity at Harvard would soon be eclipsed by an even more famous muscleman-turned-healer, Dudley Allen Sargent. A circus acrobat and weight lifter, Sargent earned an MD from Yale, teaching gymnastics when not dissecting cadavers, and went on to take over Harvard's famed Hemenway Gymnasium. There he conducted thousands of tests on the human body to perfect his training exercises, earning him the title "Grandfather of Fitness Testing." He included women in his training, one of the first to do so, and established his Sanatory Gymnasium in Cambridge, a private gym that catered to women at the Harvard Annex, which later became Radcliffe. He made the code of sportsmanship an integral part of college athletics and won the admiration of his elite students, among them Luther Gulick, as well as Theodore Roosevelt and

Henry Cabot Lodge. His invention of exercise machines with weights and pulleys was the precursor of equipment that featured variable resistance.

Other equipment went through major changes in the nineteenth century. As far back as 1772, Benjamin Franklin had extolled the use of wooden dumbbells ("I have with the use of it quickened my pulse from sixty to one hundred beats a minute," he wrote in a letter), but Windship gets credit for inventing the first plate-loaded barbell, packing the globes with iron shot (some give the nod to Triat). Any number of other weighted devices—the kettlebell, the ring bell, even the Nautical Wheel (a converted ship's wheel)—found their way into gyms. So did Indian clubs, the feared weapon of Indian soldiers, adopted by the British when they colonized the country. A hugely popular 1866 book by the American S. D. Kehoe, *The Indian Club Exercises*, was used by the U.S. Army and early baseball teams. Kehoe claimed the clubs would steady the nerves of billiard players and promised, "All are adorned with Kehoe's Missives on Muscular Christianity." The clubs were great draws at churches, which organized "swing club" socials, largely for women.

Machines became popular. Many of the contraptions look surprisingly similar to equipment in today's home gyms or health clubs, albeit with more exotic names and a touch of Rube Goldberg; the "Spalding Semi-Circle Strength Developer" was a curved half-moon bench that looked more threatening than therapeutic. D. L. Dowd's "Health Exerciser—for Brain-Workers and Sedentary People," a confusion of weighted ropes and pulleys, was "indorsed by 20,000 physicians, lawyers, clergymen and editors." There were rowing machines, home equipment ("Dr. Barnett's Improved Parlor Gymnasium"—essentially a rubber cord with handles at each end, not unlike some products sold on twenty-first-century infomercials), even a treadmill, though it was intended for animals, allowing dogs to power butter churns.

The goal of all these devices was an improved body and state of mind. But for many, vigorous health was less a product of what one did with the body than the food one put into it—or how one put food into it. None here had a mightier impact than Horace Fletcher, the Great Masticator. Comic, perhaps, when viewed a hundred years hence, he was a pioneer in the emerging field of health science and an avatar of the positive thinking that came to grip America at the century's end. Endowed with a boisterous ego and boundless energy, he circled the globe four times; managed a New Orleans opera company; excelled as an athlete, weight lifter, painter, and marksman; and settled in a palace on the Grand Canal in Venice, determined to drop his body weight that was bloated by gourmandism. He accomplished the feat by chewing food hundreds of times until it was reduced to a tasteless paste.

The twin promise of weight loss and vigor — Fletcher biked two hundred miles on his fiftieth birthday — convinced tens of thousands to give chewing its due. The practice also had its loftier goals, wedding mankind's salvation to the salivary tract: "In his assertion that thorough mastication meant going back to nature," wrote historian Harvey Green, "he implicitly criticized a civilization he thought had somehow diverted men and women from the purity that was part of life in 'primal times.'" Among his more celebrated converts were both William and Henry James. "I Fletcherize, and that's my life," the novelist brother wrote to Fletcher. "I mean it makes my life possible, and it has enormously improved my work. You ought to have a handsome percentage on every volume I sell."

The verb *Fletcherize* was coined by cereal baron John Harvey Kellogg, another of the era's nutritional zealots. As a young physician and hygienist, Kellogg had taken over the Battle Creek Sanitarium in Battle Creek, Michigan, which was owned and operated by Seventh-Day Adventists. An avid vegetarian, he rooted the cause of disease in the intestinal tract and was devoted to his enema machine, delivering large infusions of water followed by yogurt. He advocated sexual abstinence and campaigned against masturbation, which he believed caused cancer and insanity. At the "San" — as it was known — his patients would range from presidents (William Howard Taft) to aviators (Amelia Earhart); he treated George Bernard Shaw, Henry Ford, and Thomas Edison. As many as fourteen hundred people were tended by an equal number of staff. Kellogg became best known, of course, for his invention of Corn Flakes, claiming that a rival breakfast pioneer, Charles W. Post, stole the formula from his safe in the Sanitarium office. Post, an inventor and engineer, had spent nine months at the "San," hoping to cure a variety of health problems. When nothing worked, he tried Christian Science, faith healing, and positive thinking — then went on to start his own health home, LaVita Inn, where he banned tea, coffee, and physicians. Three years later he created a cereal "coffee" made from bran, wheat, and molasses, which he called Postum. The following year, 1898, he came up with Grape Nuts.

The cereal boom was merely one indication of an invigorated fit-minded America as the century drew to a close. The practice of athletics had mushroomed, especially team sports with the popularity of baseball and football. The strenuous outdoor life was given an added boost by Teddy Roosevelt. Modernity itself was on full display at the 1893 Columbian Exposition in Chicago. The Electricity Building showed the first motion pictures, while a giant Ferris wheel spun two thousand riders over the fairgrounds, though the triumph of technology was not the fair's only attraction. On the crowded midway and in a nearby nightclub, scaled-down human feats were just as likely to elicit gasps of astonishment. It was in the nightclub, the Trocadero, that America got its first glimpse of a man who would ignite a new worship of the muscled male body and all that it promised in the century to come.

CHAPTER 2

Selling the Body Beautiful, 1900–1930s

Eugen Sandow makes women faint; Bernarr Macfadden proselytizes for physical culture; Charles Atlas turns bullied scarecrows into men; Bob Hoffman builds a business with iron

THE GREAT SANDOW

It would have been hard to miss his arrival in Chicago. Before the World's Fair opened, the city was blanketed with thousands of flyers, each more fantastic than the one before. "Stands out against the background of history like some great Olympian giant, a veritable Colossus of Rhodes," one trumpeted. There had been strongmen before, but few matched his feats, and none could equal his striking features or chiseled physique. To guarantee attention, invitations were sent to some of Chicago's most prominent women, many of whom showed up for the act's opening night at the Trocadero. They were not disappointed. Silhouetted in a black-velvet box, his near-naked body dusted with white powder, the man tensed his muscles and struck classic poses that evoked Hercules and Ajax. He lifted unimaginable weights and performed his famous human dumbbell act. Afterward, a few select ladies were invited to come backstage and experience the phenomenon firsthand. As one chronicler of the social scene put it, "You were no one, really no one, my dear, unless you felt Sandow's muscles."

His name was Eugen Sandow. He was born Friedrich Wilhelm Müller in Prussia in 1867 but switched to Sandow in part to dodge the Prussian draft, in part because he dreamed of a career onstage whose performers traditionally changed their names. The son of a greengrocer, he got on poorly with his family and left home to join the circus as an acrobat. Stranded in Brussels when the circus went bankrupt, he was spotted by the famed strongman Louis Durlacher, otherwise known as "Professor Attila." Attila was so impressed by Sandow's physique and carved good looks that he took him on as his pupil and eventually lured him to England, where two wily vaudevillians, Sampson and Cyclops, were staging a much-hyped contest at London's Royal Aquarium.

Feats of strength in those days consisted of dead lifts. Sampson had hefted a weight of 2,240 pounds — an imperial ton! — or so read the barbell he raised above his head. Unbeknownst to the audience, who were invited to test the weight first, the barbell was secretly drained of its heavy sand while Sampson's emcee described the astonishing act they were about to witness. The evening of the contest, Sampson issued his usual dare, challenging anyone in the audience to match his lifts, whereupon Attila rose from his box and introduced his unlikely companion, who had come dressed in stylish evening clothes and sporting a monocle.

The crowd hooted, then fell silent when Sandow bounded onstage and ripped off his foppish costume to reveal an athletic tunic and Roman sandals. He easily matched Sampson's lifts, astonishing the audience when he raised a 220-pound barbell with a single hand. Cyclops, a burly Polish wrestler, stepped up to deprive Sandow of his prize money, twice raising a 150-pound dumbbell and a 100-pound kettlebell. As the crowd shouted, "Don't do it, you have already won the money!" Sandow easily lifted the weights — not twice but seven times.

The audience broke into thunderous applause, and Sandow's career was launched. For four years he toured British music halls, thrilling crowds while he honed his act — lifting unheard-of weights or breaking a chain locked around his fifty-two-inch chest. In what was the dawn of the age of photography, he marketed himself in gladiator poses, posed provocatively against a column, often nude except for a fig leaf. He showed off his extraordinary muscle control at Sandhurst, the elite military school; invited onstage, one audience member called feeling his muscles like "running your hand over corrugated iron." Risking what few had done before, he took his act across the Atlantic and, in 1893, appeared at New York's Casino Theater on Forty-Second Street, finishing the evening with his trademark showstopper, the so-called Tomb of Hercules. Lying on his back, he had a heavy plank laid across his chest and then arched his body into a bridge — whereupon three horses were led across.

Spectacular as the act was, Sandow enjoyed only minimal acclaim. It was early summer, and New York City was in the grip of a fierce heat wave. Few wanted to spend an evening in a hot, stuffy theater, and Sandow might have returned to Europe, poor and unknown to America, had not fate intervened with a knock on his dressing-room door. The man who entered was short and mustached. He held a contract in his hand. Burlesque crowds were well and good, he explained, but he had a much bigger audience in mind. That summer the Columbian Exposition was set to open in Chicago. When Sandow expressed skepticism and asked how he had arranged it, the man seemed taken aback. "Don't you know who I am?" he exclaimed. "I'm Florenz Ziegfeld!"

He was the twenty-six-year-old son of Florenz Ziegfeld Sr., the concert-hall impresario, and he was on a mission. The family owned the Trocadero Theater in Chicago, where profits had been less than stellar. Dispatched by his father to recruit significant acts in Europe, notably the great German conductor Hans von Bulow, the young Ziegfeld came back with the "Bulow Military Band" and a trio of Swiss mountaineers who yodeled and clogged. Lambasted by his father, Ziegfeld was determined to make a hit of his New York talent search—and he did. It was Ziegfeld who wrote the outrageous flyers, Ziegfeld who invited the city's society women, Ziegfeld who had Sandow dusted with white powder and then placed in a black-velvet cabinet. The act proved such a sensation that, once the Columbian Exposition closed, he launched Sandow on a yearlong tour of U.S. cities that would make both men famous.

Sex played a big part. It became a regular part of the show that paying patrons were invited backstage to feel his rock-hard muscles, an experience so shocking that women were known to faint. It is unlikely that any of these intimate sessions resulted in more than erotic groping. Sandow was no philanderer, not then anyway. Halfway through the tour he married a woman named Blanche Baker, a photographer's assistant. Ziegfeld, his star's irrepressible keeper, did his best to quash word of the marriage, just as he attempted to repress even worse rumors—Sandow's relationship with the act's male musical conductor, classical pianist Martinus Sieveking. There was little to document the exact nature of their relationship, but plenty of room for conjecture. Arriving in New York, the two shared an apartment where a visiting reporter for the *New York Journal* described Sieveking stripped of his shirt, ogling Sandow's muscles.

Sandow's American tour was an unprecedented triumph. Proclaiming himself "the World's Most Perfect Man," and with Ziegfeld churning the publicity machine, he made headlines in every city he visited. He arrived with great fanfare, staying in luxury suites in plush hotels. Doctors and reporters were encouraged to pound his abdomen during strolls through the audience. In New York the great photographer Napoleon Sarony produced an album of portraits that became classics of early physique photography. He wrestled a lion in Golden Gate Park (albeit a muzzled one with gloved paws). He visited Thomas Alva Edison in West Orange, New Jersey, where the inventor was perfecting his Kinetoscope using a crude loop of celluloid film. The resultant "motion picture" of Sandow lifting weights thrilled viewers crowded into peephole-like "parlors."

Sandow had already made his name as bodybuilding's greatest showman, but more was to come. Back in England he turned to business. He created *Sandow's Magazine*, which promoted exercise for both men and women. He opened his first Institute of Physical Culture. Unlike the more proletarian working-class gyms, Sandow's was an upscale operation that resembled a rich, wood-paneled Victorian club with individual carpets that marked each exercise station. Women were encouraged to come, though in keeping with prevailing rules of modesty, their exercise area was curtained off to ensure privacy.

He invented and marketed equipment. He promoted the "curative" powers of exercise—in particular his own methods. In 1897 he published a book, *Strength and How to Obtain It*, which included a foldout chart of exercises to be hung on a wall. The book was a huge best seller and was mentioned in James Joyce's *Ulysses* in the catalog of books in Leopold Bloom's library. As pointed out by one Joyce scholar, Bloom turns to Sandow's exercise regime whenever he faces self-doubt or failure. Sandow was the obvious model of a young prizefighter, Sandel, in the Jack London story "A Piece of Streak." He started a magazine called *Physical Culture*, which included articles by Frederick Jane (the author of the maritime bible, *All the World's Fighting Ships*) and P. G. Wodehouse. He had a serious admirer in Sir Arthur Conan Doyle.

Doyle, a huge man at six-foot-four and weighing more than 230 pounds, worshipped physical strength and imbued Sherlock Holmes with impressive feats (in "The Speckled Band," he straightens an iron poker after the giant Dr. Grimsby Rowlett bends it double to intimidate the detective). Doyle wrote the introduction to two of Sandow's books and was on the judging panel for Sandow's Great Competition – the much-publicized contest he staged in 1901 in Royal Albert Hall. Among the many celebrities who endorsed Sandow's work, his exercise system, and its curative powers was none other than England's King George V, who issued a royal warrant that named Sandow his personal "Professor of Scientific and Physical Culture." Likely the title was more honorific than practical, but Sandow's onetime publicity hound, Florenz Ziegfeld, would have relished the hype.

During the first two decades of the twentieth century, Sandow kept furiously busy. He appeared in competitions; he had a plaster cast made of his body. He toured Australia and Africa; he returned to America for a twelve-month series of exhibitions, appearing at Harvard College and the Hemenway Gymnasium, where Dudley Sargent called him "the most perfectly developed man the world has ever seen." In gratitude Sandow presented him with the cast of his body, its value priceless.

His name remained legend, but Sandow's own fortunes faded. His once-iron muscles showed the slack of age. Competing magazines forced him to end his publishing career. His wife, Blanche, long bitter over his rumored affairs, refused to speak to him, as did one of his daughters. When Sandow died in 1925, Blanche had him buried in a rustic cemetery at Putney Vale, near London, and barred the erection of a grave marker.

The exact cause of Sandow's death remains a subject of controversy. News reports had him dying of a burst blood vessel in his brain after heroically and single-handedly lifting a car from a ditch to save its trapped occupant. Further investigation made that claim seem far-fetched. The supposed auto accident was years before; he was reputedly ill; no man, even the great Sandow, could have hoisted a one-ton car.

Almost a century after his death, his grave remains unmarked at Putney Vale. The magnificent plaster cast presented to Sargent at Harvard, after years of exhibit, was taken down and stored, then simply vanished.

THE FATHER OF PHYSICAL CULTURE

Sandow had many admirers and not a few imitators. The most notorious was Bernarr Macfadden, who was in Chicago the summer of the Columbian Exposition. Like tens of thousands, he was mesmerized by Sandow's strongman poses. Macfadden then was twenty-five, a year younger than

Sandow and the mere slip of a man compared to the mighty Prussian. At five-foot-six and 145 pounds, he was anything but overwhelming in size. What he had was tenacious ambition and a survivor's instinct for turning circumstance in his favor. Sandow's trick with white powder and a black-velvet background was quickly filed away in his memory. It would not be the last idea he would borrow from Sandow.

Macfadden had grown up dirt-poor in the tiny Ozark town of Mill Springs, Missouri. It was not a happy childhood. His rough, hard-drinking father died from an alcoholic seizure; not long after Macfadden's mother moved the family to St. Louis. Sick and destitute, she sent Bernard — the name he was born with — to a boarding school, then had him shipped to a cheap hotel in Illinois, where the nine-year-old worked one-hundred-hour weeks emptying chamber pots and scrubbing floors. His mother died soon after, and there followed grueling work on a farm with a foster father — transformative for Macfadden, who seized on the great outdoors as the ideal place to strengthen his body. The farmer, a quarrelsome cheapskate, finally made life intolerable, and Macfadden hopped a train to St. Louis to live with relatives and stumbled on a gymnasium filled with German immigrants — strapping athletic specimens who had imported their home country's turnverein. Too poor to join, he bought dumbbells. He discovered the 1879 best seller *How to Get Strong and How to Stay So* by William Blaikie, a strongman protégé of Sargent who compared the sad state of America's youth with the robust English lads in *Tom Brown's School Days*. He promoted boxing bouts and became a champion wrestler, defeating much bigger men in grueling matches. He landed a job as physical director at a private boys' school, the Marmaduke Military Academy, and tossed off an eighty-thousand-word novel, *The Athlete's Conquest*, in his spare time. School over, on the prowl for novelty and adventure, he took the train to Chicago.

He bankrolled his stay there by demonstrating the Whitely Exerciser, a wall-mounted contraption of ropes and pulleys that was invented by a friend, Alexander Whitely. The fair over, he headed to New York City with fifty dollars in his pocket, wrote articles, peddled the Exerciser, invented his own device (which was remarkably similar), and promoted a personal-trainer business with the made-up title of "professor." Long a fanatic about healthy food and natural healing (he had once cured an incipient bout of pneumonia by fasting on a few daily pieces of fruit), he starved himself down to 135 pounds for publicity photos and gave it all up for a tour of England, following in Sandow's footsteps and apparently filching the name of his institute, because back in New York he started a magazine called *Physical Culture*.

The first issue came out in March 1899 and sold for five cents. It was published out of a small room in a real-estate office near the Brooklyn Bridge. The slim twenty-page magazine was little more than a sales catalog for Macfadden's exerciser. The entire contents of the magazine were written by Macfadden, including the articles with women's bylines. The photos were all bodybuilding poses – of Macfadden. The magazine had a single employee – Macfadden. The cover – which bore the phrase "Weakness Is a Crime. Don't Be a Criminal." – depicted a muscular young man in classical poses identified as "Professor Macfadden."

Within five years the magazine had moved to spacious new offices, had fifty employees, and was selling one hundred thousand copies. What set *Physical Culture* apart from its competition – between 1830 and 1890, eighty-five health magazines were started in the United States – were three things, according to Mark Adams, the author of a Macfadden biography: "He freely used celebrities, he sought women readers as well as men, and he seasoned every issue with a healthy dose of sex."

Sex got the most attention. Macfadden was years – decades – ahead of his time. Articles such as "What a Young Woman Ought to Know" incensed prudish critics but were not unlike cover lines in a modern-day *Cosmopolitan*. Reputing Victorian notions of female frailty, he promoted feminine strength and muscular beauty, often with an eye toward erotic appeal. In a separate magazine for women called *Beauty and Health*, he ran group photos of women in scanty attire, often in the company of men who wore even less. Just as provocative were his tirades against the medical establishment. He lambasted the doctors who had fed President McKinley a slice of bread dipped in beef juice soon after McKinley was shot (a 2011 book excoriated McKinley's doctors for far worse lapses). He attacked the evils of vaccination (as a boy Macfadden had nearly died after being scratched with live small pox vaccine). He fumed against the evils of fat, meat, white bread, sugar, and excess calories. He offered to cure, free of charge and with natural healing, any patients abandoned by their ignorant doctors.

The magazine prospered, encouraging Macfadden, who rarely needed encouragement, to expand his titles. He would eventually publish dozens of magazines, among them *True Confessions* and *True Story*, whose circulation topped one and a half million in 1925. At its peak Macfadden's publishing empire was so widespread that its combined circulation was well over seven million, topping that of both William Randolph Hearst and Henry Luce. His most sensational title was the *Graphic*, quickly dubbed the "Porno-Graphic," a forerunner of today's tabloids, which offered lurid reports on crime, sex, and scandal. Printed on hot-pink paper, it specialized in first-person headline shockers—"We Faced Death Together in the Flames," "I Am the Mother of My Sister's Son"—and reports on serious news that went beyond, way beyond, yellow journalism. Sacco and Vanzetti's execution ran under the all-caps "ROASTED ALIVE!" The *Graphic* was also where Walter Winchell and Ed Sullivan first earned their reporting chops as regular columnists.

But it was fitness that truly obsessed Macfadden. Taking another cue from Sandow, he staged the "Physical Fitness Competition," promoting it for months in *Physical Culture* and with thousands of posters plastered around Manhattan. The extravaganza, featuring a separate contest for women, was a huge success. It was the even bigger sequel, his "Physical Culture Show," that prompted his first run-in with blue-nose crusader Anthony Comstock. Arrested for lewd posters and let off with a suspended sentence, he got nabbed again by Comstock for the *Physical Culture* feature that depicted the dangers of venereal disease, a subject that was rarely discussed openly. Convicted and sentenced to two years in jail, he was saved by the last-minute intervention of President Taft.

The near escape did nothing to stem his furious energy or output during the subsequent years. He opened restaurants and sold exercise equipment and wrote books. His crowning achievement was a twenty-nine-hundred-page five-volume encyclopedia that addressed every subject from exercise to nutrition, from medical quackery to sexual relations. On an eighteen-hundred-acre tract of New Jersey land, he built his utopia—Physical Culture City. Enticed by the success of the cereal barons Kellogg and Post in Battle Creek, Michigan, he opened a "Macfadden Sanatorium" there—a luxury mansion with pools, baths, and a gym. The celebrated treatment—for just about any ailment—was a ten-day fast followed by a milk diet that required drinking eight quarts a day. True believers included novelist Upton Sinclair, who came to recover from the rigors of writing *The Jungle* and dedicated his next novel, *Samuel the Seeker*, to Macfadden. He took his act to Chicago and opened the "Macfadden Healthatorium" in an inspiring South Side building.

When things looked bleak — his first wife divorced him, legal expenses soared — he sold his properties, entrusted his publishing interests to colleagues, and headed to England, where, with typical brazen hype, he staged a nationwide contest to discover "Great Britain's perfect woman." The winner, whom Macfadden personally inspected, along with all finalists, was a nineteen-year-old champion swimmer, Mary Williamson, whom he married. Together they toured England as "the world's most perfectly developed couple." Their act climaxed with Mary climbing atop a seven-foot platform and jumping on Macfadden's chest. They returned on the *Lusitania*, and she promptly bore him the first of a brood whom he named Berwyn, Beulah, Beverly, Braunda, Brewster, Brynece, and Byron.

Everything he did was marked by extremes. He was fanatic about exercise — he walked six miles to work barefoot and did five hundred morning sit-ups — and no less rabid in matters of health, demonizing doctors for failing to promote his "natural" cure for every ailment known to man, from bad eyesight to baldness. Many of his beliefs were dubious at best: nightmares, he insisted, were caused by bad digestion; all disease was caused by impure blood. Some of his practices were worse: when his firstborn weighed in at a disappointing five pounds, he submerged the baby in ice-cold water to stimulate growth. Yet he was far ahead of his times in the stock he put in sex education. He waged war against prudery and ignorance. The establishment — the food industry, traditional medicine, church groups — did what they could to dismiss him. *Time* branded him a "kook" and a "charlatan," and certainly he was full of contradictions. Though he campaigned against nicotine and medical quackery, the pages of the *Graphic* were filled with ads for cigarettes and sorcerers' nostrums. He preached the sanctity of marriage — yet fathered a child with his secretary at Physical Culture City.

No matter: he elevated the pursuit of health and fitness to a place where they had never been before. He had a talent for brazen self-promotion and headline stunts that dwarfed his rivals in publishing. Who but Macfadden would have tapped First Lady Eleanor Roosevelt to guest-edit his new magazine for babies? (She accepted.) Who but

Macfadden would have donned a football helmet and hockey kneepads for a parachute jump to mark his seventieth birthday? (He did jumps every year thereafter, until age eighty.) Who but Macfadden, age seventy-two, would have run for a Senate seat from Florida? (He very nearly won a spot in the Democratic runoff.)

His success and notoriety were partly a result of his full-tilt grandstanding—and partly reflective of the times. The early decades of the twentieth century marked a watershed when it came to views of the body. The world had begun to shed Victorian restraints and the notion of "respectability." The new field of psychology, especially the work of Sigmund Freud, urged the elimination of guilt and shame; a fuller understanding of the mind's working promised freedom from social stigma. For Macfadden, all sense of self started and ended with the human body. He was tagged "Body Love Macfadden" in *Time*, which meant it pejoratively. But for Macfadden and his mass of followers, the term was the highest praise.

"A strong and beautiful body has become a thing of honor and glory," he wrote in 1924 in the introduction to one of his cookbooks, "and the proper feeding of the body a duty recognized and a pleasure to be enjoyed by all." He raised cultivation of the body to the level of a virtual religion. His admonition—"Weakness is a crime; don't be a criminal"—was preceded by "Sickness is a sin; don't be a sinner."

Ultimately, his rabid doctrines and whitewash of nonbelievers did not serve him well. His declining years were just that—a descent into poverty and insignificance. A big believer in selective breeding and racial nationalism, he became enamored of Mussolini. In old age he seemed more a fool than a prophet. At seventy-nine he took a forty-year-old bride, a vivacious Texan who balked when he insisted she sew his name onto the rear of her white tights for a parachute jump—and soon divorced him. Mary penned a torrid if entertaining exposé of their marriage, *Dumbbells and Carrot Strips*, which she dedicated "particularly to those merciful doctors ever ready to reduce the pain of childbirth." Macfadden, meanwhile, was jailed for nonpayment of debt and died after being discovered unconscious in a seedy Jersey City hotel, likely from jaundice and dehydration. His greatest discovery and prodigy would far outstrip him in the arena of public opinion, though the man had none of Macfadden's verve, none of his entrepreneurial derring-do, none of his messianic outrage. What he had was a magnificent chest, perfectly proportioned limbs, and an easy manner that suggested anyone, with a modicum of effort and determination, could be just like him.

"I WANT TO MAKE A MAN OUT OF YOU!"

Charles Atlas was born in the tiny town of Acri in southern Italy. He arrived with his parents at Ellis Island in 1903 at age ten. His name was Angelo Siciliano, and he spoke not a word of English.

He did not look like much, either. Skinny and slope shouldered, feeble and often ill, he was picked on by bullies in the Brooklyn neighborhood where his mother had settled. His father had taken one look at America and gone back home, leaving the young boy in the hands of an uncle, who himself beat him when Angelo did not fight back.

According to the Atlas legend—and supported by oft-repeated personal testimony—three events served to turn things around. When Angelo visited Coney Island Beach in the company of a girl, a hunky lifeguard kicked sand in his face. The girl rolled her eyes, while Angelo, humiliated, swore revenge. On a school trip to the Brooklyn Museum, he stared stupefied at the muscled statues of Hercules, Apollo, and Zeus. He went home and devised a series of makeshift weights, ropes, and elastic grips to build up his body. The results were disappointing. On a visit to the Bronx Zoo, he watched a lion stretch and had an epiphany. "Does this old gentleman have any barbells, any exercisers?" he would later recall. "And it came over me . . . He's been pitting one muscle against another!"

He threw out his equipment. He struck poses and flexed his muscles, using what would later be known as isometric opposition. The results, after much work, were impressive. On the beach one day, an astounded friend exclaimed, "You look like that statue of Atlas on top of the Atlas Hotel!" Several years later, he legally changed his name, adding Charles from his nickname, "Charlie."

He took a five-dollar-a-week job as a janitor and strongman at the Coney Island sideshow, where he lay on a bed of nails and urged men from the audience to stand on his stomach. On the beach one day, he was spotted by an artist who asked him to pose, launching his career as a sculptor's model. By the time he was twenty-five, Atlas—or his facsimile—was everywhere: he was George Washington in Washington Square Park, Civic Virtue in Queens Borough Hall, Alexander Hamilton in the nation's capital. Socialite sculptress Gloria Vanderbilt, watching Atlas disrobe, exclaimed, "He's a knockout!"

Macfadden was equally impressed. Following Atlas's second triumph at the "World's Most Perfectly Developed Man" competition, he called a halt to all future contests, griping Atlas would win every year. Their paths would cross only briefly thereafter—though once with great consequence. After Atlas's triumph, Macfadden tapped a bodybuilder and marketing maven at *Physical Culture* named Frederick W. Tilney to direct a movie starring Atlas. It was Tilney's suggestion that he and Atlas team up to offer a mail-order course. Perhaps it was "merely remarkable coincidence," as Macfadden's biographer suggests, that the first several years of Atlas's mail-order course included a sixty-four-page booklet titled *Secrets of Muscular Power and Beauty*—virtually identical to Macfadden's 1906 treatise, *Muscular Power and Beauty*, which was all about isometric exercise. Perhaps it was coincidence again that Atlas's ads in *Physical Culture* identified him first as "Prof. Chas Atlas."

What is indisputable is that Atlas's subsequent success would likely not have happened were it not for another Charles—Charles Roman. Atlas had an extraordinary body but no head for business. Ending his partnership with Tilney, he elected to go it solo, and his mail-order company took a belly flop. It was saved by a twenty-one-year-old copywriter fresh out of New York University to whom Atlas handed his advertising account. The ads so impressed Atlas that he offered Roman half the company if Roman would run it. Roman did, for the next forty years.

It was Roman who coined the term *Dynamic Tension*. It was Roman who wrote all the Atlas ads, from the "Hey, Skinny!" strips to the "97-Pound Weakling" and "The Insult That Made a Man Out of Mac" series. Theirs was a partnership of muscle and marketing that perfectly exploited the mood of the country. The ads went straight to the male psyche. They preyed on every man's insecurity—that he was not "man enough" to defend his girl at the beach. At a time when the nation was reeling from the 1929 stock market crash and its aftermath, Atlas's ads promised to restore a million battered male egos.

The ad campaigns marked a dramatic new turn in the appeal of fitness. Previously, exercise had been the habit of a few, motivated by health first, with vanity a distant second. Many gaped at the muscle-bound Sandows, but few saw them as real-life idols. Roman's ads heralded a new view of a man's body—as a measurement, quite literally, of success. This was a time when millions migrated from rural America to cities and sterile look-alike offices. Making an impression counted. It was why Dale Carnegie's *How to Win Friends and Influence People* turned into a publishing phenomenon. But whereas Carnegie preached advancement through social skills, Atlas evangelized for the body beautiful.

Roman's ads were also emblematic of a new era in advertising, if not an important influence on it. The first few decades of the twentieth century marked a dramatic boom for an industry beginning to flex its own muscle. It was coming to exert a major force in the culture, and its leaders knew it. *The J. Walter Thompson Book*, a pamphlet to propagandize the advertising agency, offered this bit of self-promotion: "Advertising is *revolutionary*. Its tendency is to overturn preconceived notions, to set new ideas spinning through the reader's brain, to induce something that they never did before. It is a form of progress, and it interests only progressive people."

Advertisers saw themselves as a "civilizing" influence on the untold millions who still clung to Victorian ideals. The transition from Puritanism to hedonism meant a new emphasis on freedom from restraint, a coddling of the revitalized human body. With that attention, however, came anxiety and fear—which the admen were quick to exploit. Health and cleanliness required upkeep: deodorant and talcum powders and skin creams and breath fresheners. The healthy body was the groomed body; shaving was a triumph of the civilized world, "from Boston to Bombay," trumpeted an ad for Gillette razors.

In this new world so worshipful of the clean, coiffed gentleman, Charles Atlas was the perfect upstanding specimen—not a freak of nature from the fringe circuses and dingy sideshows. He was never the strongest man on the planet. He did not promote the kind of bulging muscles that made women swoon (though his proportions were deemed so ideal that the actual dimensions would be buried in a time capsule at Oglethorpe University, along with a tiny statuette). What set him apart were his steady demeanor and perfect proportions. "His smooth 'aesthetic' poses evoking classical sculpture set the standard for the 'ideal human body' of the 1920s and 1930s," noted Donald J. Mrozek in *Sport and American Life*. "[It was] a standard emphasizing personal grace and suggesting ease, quiet confidence and contentment."

Exercise was key, but the body also had to be nurtured. It required monitoring and coaching. In his many brochures, Atlas wrote frequently about the importance of posture and the proper way to sleep and rise ("Get up immediately on awakening in the morning. . . . Don't dilly-dally. GET UP!") He advocated bathing the genital organs every morning in cold water and urged rubbing olive oil into the scalp. He penned long treatises on various maladies, and his company published books on everything from child rearing to relationship advice. Like Macfadden, he tied marital success to a robust sense of well-being. "The lack of glorious vigorous health," he noted, "would prove to be, if the divorce records were analyzed, the most common reason why so many marriages 'crack up.'"

There was, of course, a dark side to the ads that Roman concocted, one that feasted on anxiety and pools of insecurity. "What Kind of Man Are You?" demanded a typical ad for *Muscular Power and Beauty*. "Look Yourself in the Mirror. Be a Man — Not a Manikin." "Let Me Prove That I Can Make YOU a New Man!" he declared with a stern look and jabbing finger.

Whether to the carrot or the stick, readers responded. Mail deluged the company offices on Eighth Avenue. At its peak Atlas had twenty-nine women opening letters and taking checks for Dynamic Tension. Ads in more than four hundred comic books and magazines brought in forty thousand recruits each year. The personal response was key: his lessons took the form of letters signed by the man himself: "Yours for Health and Strength" or "Yours in Perfect Manhood" or, during World War II, "Yours for Lasting Peace." Long before personal trainers, Atlas tried to create an intimate bond with his "students." That the exercises could be performed alone at home, without risk of embarrassment at a YMCA or gym, was part of their appeal.

In person Atlas was a charming spokesman. He rarely lost his temper. A lone documented lapse was when he was again called before the Federal Trade Commission (FTC) in 1939 to defend his strength-building system. "What's the matter with those fellows in Washington," he fumed to reporters before the commission exonerated him for the third time of all charges. "I'm doing the cleanest job of any man living today."

And likely he was. His values were curiously old-fashioned, even quaint. He was an active promoter of the Boy Scouts. Asked for advice, he would say, "Live clean, think clean and don't go to burlesque shows." Unlike Roman, who spent his growing fortune on luxury cars, yachts, and private planes, he had few indulgences beyond a taste for white double-breasted suits. He lived in a four-room fifth-floor walkup apartment in Brooklyn with his two children and wife, Margaret, to whom he was singularly devoted. The family retreat was a modest home at Point Lookout on Long Island.

Was he too good to be true? Not according to Robert Ripley of *Ripley's Believe It or Not*, a friend of Atlas who once saw him dive into the surf off Coney Island and rescue a boat and its foundering occupants. Certainly, Atlas enjoyed the limelight. He loved to pose with celebrities—trading jibes with boxing champions Max Baer and Joe Louis. He delighted in publicity stunts (most of them engineered by Roman): towing a 145,000-pound locomotive along a Queens railroad track; entertaining inmates at Sing-Sing (prompting the headline "Man Breaks Bars at Sing-Sing—Thousands Cheer, None Escape"). He was a guest on Jack Dempsey's radio program; he tore telephone books in half for visiting columnists who dropped by for amusing copy. But he never alienated his public. If not humble, he was never arrogant, never a rabid missionary.

There is some question about his honesty. Not a few have disputed the claim that his miraculous physique was achieved entirely through Dynamic Tension. Joe Weider, the Canadian bodybuilder and future publishing magnate, liked to tell of an encounter at the New York Athletic Club when Atlas told him a 100-pound barbell was too heavy to ship and advised: "'Joe, I just send a course and some pictures and I make so much more money than you do. You should do that, too.' In my heart," said Weider, "I knew that using weights was greatly superior to dynamic tension, but I didn't want to argue with him." Several weight lifters were more emphatic. The famed Bill Pearl stated flatly: "Charles Atlas built his body primarily through weight training and not through Dynamic Tension." The most infamous challenge to Atlas came from a man who had good reason to question his methods; he had made his fortune from barbells. In testimony before the FTC, where he had had to answer a complaint charging unfair business practices, he called Atlas's system "Dynamic Hooey."

BULLY OF THE IRON GAME

Bob Hoffman is one of the legends of the "Iron Game"—the name given to the practice of hefting dumbbells and barbells to build muscles. At the time of the FTC hearings, 1936, Hoffman was enjoying unprecedented success as a weight lifter, fitness promoter, and barbell manufacturer. He ran all his activities out of York, Pennsylvania, a small city known mostly for building air conditioners, motorcycles, caskets, and dentures. Hoffman himself had started an oil-burner business there with the son of a local plumber. A rabid salesman, he made the company hugely profitable and roused his employees to join in his favorite activity: weight training.

He was a big man, six-foot-three, slender but athletic. He had grown up on a 640-acre farm in Georgia, where—in yet another variation of the sick-turned-mighty myth—he almost died of typhoid fever caused by drinking contaminated water. He found his first dumbbell in a country dump. He was a much-decorated soldier during World War I, earning three Croix de Guerres from France and a Purple Heart. Ever ready to puff up his chest, he returned from war and began his weight-training career with the declaration, "Whatever I take up, I become a champion." He packed pounds onto his body and, true to his word, won the 1927 United States Heavyweight Championship (he was also the only competitor in his weight class). He installed a weight-training platform in the middle of his oil-burner factory, where, each afternoon at 4:30, he led his employees in a two-hour workout session.

The results were astonishing. Identified by their T-shirts emblazoned with "The York Oil Burner Athletic Club" but known more informally as "the York Gang," the group would grow to include twenty-five champion bodybuilders and weight lifters, among them the great John Grimek. The year of the FTC hearing, a York-based team headed for Hitler's much-ballyhooed Berlin Olympics, placing a respectable if disappointing third behind Germany and Egypt. Hoffman, crushed, was redeemed a decade later, in 1946, when the United States captured its first world championship with four of the six lifters employed by what had then become the York Barbell Company.

In personality Hoffman was a lot closer to Macfadden than Atlas. Brash, abrasive, a brazen self-promoter, he assumed the title of "the World's Healthiest Man," claiming never to have had a cold or suffered a headache. He feuded with competitors and often made claims that his own biographer, John Fair, dismissed as "delusions of grandeur." Unlike Macfadden, a serial monogamist (with a few exceptions), and Atlas, the family man, Hoffman was a lifelong womanizer and proud of it. He had a common-law wife, Alda, twenty years his junior, but never let that slow him down. "The only thing she faults me for," he confided to friend and heavyweight lifter Terry Todd, "is what she calls being unfaithful. Unfaithful! Look at it this way—I've been seeing the same four women—not counting Alda—for over twenty-five years, at least once a week when I'm in town. *The same four women!* If that's not being faithful, I don't know what faithful means."

Amused by his "Jovean ability to rationalize," Todd was quick to point out Hoffman's many achievements. He was the coach of the U.S. Olympic weightlifting team in every Games from 1948 to 1968. His York lifters won the team trophy in the U.S. Weightlifting Championships an incredible forty-eight times. He published *Strength and Health*, which became the preeminent magazine for anyone who cared about exercise and nutrition. He wrote fifty-odd books. He was a major late-life philanthropist, who became obsessed with the sport of softball and sank two hundred thousand dollars into renovating a Minor League Baseball stadium, christening it the Bob Hoffman Softball Complex. His money, an estimated fifteen million dollars in 1977, derived from diversified interests: York County real estate, two foundries, a screw company. The bulk, however, came from exercise equipment and his miraculous food supplement, Bob Hoffman's Hi-Proteen Powder.

Stories vary as to how he came up with the powder. One ascribed the invention to an early obsession with soybeans and dinners at Chinese restaurants. Another traced the tale to a York machinist, Joe Park, who had gotten the recipe from a Chicago gym where he trained, a version that had Hoffman mixing an unpalatable brew of soybean liquid with a canoe paddle and adding sweet chocolate from Hershey. Having previously touted "plain simple food" as the meal of champions, Hoffman had some explaining to do, and soon the pages of *Strength and Health* were filled with articles on nutrition, most citing "soil depletion" as reason for the update. It helped that bodybuilders, with their fabulous sculpted muscles, were suddenly gaining new attention, notably the husky Park, who had won his Mr. America, Mr. World, and Mr. Universe titles after popping hundreds of Protamin tablets. Hoffman, of course, was their biggest proponent. "I almost live on Hi-Proteen," declared Hoffman, who liked to mix the powder into a shake with milk, bananas, honey, and peanut butter. "Many days I take nothing else."

The powder or pills were easily transportable, and Hoffman had high hopes that they would help lead his team to victory in the 1954 Vienna Olympics, which was looming as a defining event in the Cold War. The early fifties had grown into a tense showdown between the rival nuclear superpowers. Who would rule space? Who had the bigger missiles to lob across oceans? Who, reduced to more human scale, could outlift whom? Recently, Soviet lifters had been embarrassing their American counterparts in competition, but Hoffman, employing Cold War terminology, called Hi-Proteen "our secret weapon."

To his chagrin, the Soviets walked away with a 29–23 win, and Hoffman returned Stateside, frustrated but vowing revenge, the means for which would soon be supplied by the U.S. team doctor, John Ziegler. Ziegler was a colorful character, a big man and fan of the Old West, who often dressed in western garb and had friends call him "Tex" or "Montana Jack." After recovering from horrific injuries in the Pacific during World War II, he had earned a medical degree and began treating the handicapped and burn patients with testosterone, which he got from CIBA pharmaceuticals. Looking for healthier specimens on whom to test the experimental shots, he hooked up with York. In Vienna he watched the Soviet men hoist their astonishing weights and suspected something fishy, especially since so many had outsized, hairy bodies. Luring his counterpart, the Soviet team physician, to a local tavern, he plied the doctor with vodka and soon learned the truth: Soviet lifters had been building their bulk with testosterone.

Back home Ziegler began administering testosterone shots to select York weight lifters. The results were negligible and came with side effects, but Ziegler kept tinkering, and, in 1958, CIBA unleashed a drug that rocked the sports world: Dianabol (methandrostenolone), one of the first anabolic steroids. Hoffman immediately tried the new pink pills on his men, and the results were stunning. By the early 1960s, the York lifters had grown as big and strong as Ajax. A few months on Dianabol added a hundred pounds to some lifts. For a while Hoffman downplayed the drug's role, stressing instead a new training protocol called "isometric contraction," which involved pushing and pulling on an immovable bar. But it was merely a sideshow. Drugs were the key, and in 1967 *Track and Field News* called anabolic steroids the "breakfast of champions."

In *Strength and Health* Hoffman began to temper his earlier enthusiasm with caution. Ziegler himself grew wary of steroid abuse, then fed up. In 1967 he left York, eventually dying from a damaged heart that he claimed was caused by his great misguided experiment. "I wish I'd never heard of anabolic steroids," he warned in a tape-recorded message before his death. "These kids don't realize the terrible price they are going to pay!"

Hoffman had other troubles. He was busier than ever, promoting the hugely successful Hi-Proteen Powder, writing books and articles, running around the country. But York itself was rocked by dissension and not a few defections. The Internal Revenue Service charged Hoffman with hiding income and slapped him with a $359,615 bill for unpaid taxes. Hoffman settled for considerably less, but the bad publicity fueled attacks from other enemies, most notably Joe Weider. In a series of articles in his new magazine, *Mr. America*, Weider tagged Hoffman a bully and womanizer, ridiculed his philanthropy, and charged him with "fixing" physique contests. Hoffman had even choicer words; he called Weider a "rat," a "skunk," and a "jackal."

The feud was both personal and philosophical. Hoffman was a firm believer in muscles serving a purpose—enhancing sports performance among athletes and, most blatantly, lifting iron. Big muscles counted for nothing if they could not win grueling contests on the world stage. Weider belonged in an opposite camp: muscles were all about physique and show. This great schism—between weight lifters and bodybuilders—fractured the world of weight training, and it made Hoffman furious. In the midfifties he heaped increasing scorn on what he tagged in *Strength and Health* as a "cult" and "boobybuilders."

"A boobybuilder," went one of his articles, "is usually a young man who has nothing better to do with his time than to spend four or five hours a day in a smelly gym doing bench presses and curls and squats and lat pulley exercises. He usually wears his hair long and frequently gilds the lily by having it waved. He is supremely concerned with big lats, big pex, big delts, and flapping triceps. . . . Athletic fitness and muscular coordination and superb health are completely meaningless to him."

Weider, sued for eight hundred thousand dollars. Hoffman counterclaimed, charging malicious conspiracy and character defamation, and in 1962 the case of the bitch-slapping musclemen/publishers went to court.

Hoffman's earlier legal wrangle with Atlas had ended as mostly a draw. In front of the FTC commissioners, he had stood upside down on his thumbs to prove the value of barbells. Impressed but not convinced, the FTC sent Hoffman off with a warning not to disparage Atlas again. He anticipated a more clear-cut victory with Weider, and the U.S. district court in Harrisburg did not disappoint. In 1962 it found Hoffman not guilty and awarded him thirty thousand dollars. Years later, on appeal, after much costly litigation, the amount was reduced to one dollar, since Hoffman had not proved monetary loss. It was another setback in Hoffman's slow demise.

Age was a primary factor. Though still proclaiming himself "the World's Healthiest Man," he began suffering a series of physical ailments that would culminate in heart bypass surgery at age seventy-nine. Ever the spin master, Hoffman tried turning the near-death experience to his own benefit. "In my eightieth year," he boasted, "I was able to withstand an operation that would have turned an ordinary older man into a vegetable."

But long before death claimed him, there were other troubles. The York defections undermined the company, which, after its heyday during the late fifties and sixties, had begun to lose traction. Competition was everywhere, and Hoffman was forced to sell off titles from his stable of magazines. Most significantly, the core appeal of York had started to weaken. It had built its stock on a population of the urban disenfranchised, men who had found themselves lost in the great melting pot. Getting strong was a way to assert their identity. But as the century wore on, the immigrant phenomenon had faded. Whereas the early York Gang featured Bulgarians, Slavs, Greeks, and Turks, increasingly the new recruits had American-sounding names. York was very much an East Coast urban phenomenon, a magnet for displaced souls who found comfort in bigger bodies. On the West Coast, on the sunny beaches of California, a very different group had begun to flaunt their sculpted muscles. The attention they would grab, and their accomplishments, would radically alter the direction of fitness.

CHAPTER 3

America Shapes Up, 1930s–1950s

Fun in the sand; Vic Tanny and Jack LaLanne spiff up gyms; Bonnie Prudden, "the First Lady of Fitness Fashion," shocks the president

MUSCLE BEACH

If Bob Hoffman was any indication, there was much to suspect in the temper and drive of the musclemen. The York Gang espoused healthy living, but many doped themselves with steroids and supplements. They lived life to the sound track of grunting lifts and the thud of dumbbells dropped on the gym floor. It did not look like a lot of fun, which was all too obvious in the pictures; as often as not, photos of Hoffman and many disciples show tensed figures, muscles flexed, often with grim, clenched expressions.

The archives of Muscle Beach tell a different story altogether. Here, on the sunny sands of Santa Monica Beach, the men (and women!) are smiling and happy. Stacked on top of each other in human pyramids, they beam with delight. Flung over the sand in daring tosses, they are captured in thrilling midair swan dives. Whereas the York Gang mostly posed singly, the denizens of Muscle Beach gather in groups, a mutual admiration society, arms wrapped around one another, smiling into the camera as if to say, "Look at the fun we're having! Come join us!" It was this sense of shared exuberance, a revel in the pleasures of a vibrant life — their bodies a mere means to an end and not the compulsive goal — that made Muscle Beach such a special phenomenon and a mecca for athletes and bodybuilders.

The phenomenon had started back in the 1930s when a handful of gymnasts and elite athletes started hanging out on the Santa Monica sand to practice hand balances and tumbling. It was a lively spectacle and soon drew crowds of onlookers. A tumbling platform was built, courtesy of the Works Progress Administration, which added equipment. In 1937 the city of Santa Monica installed a twenty-four-by-eighty-foot wooden platform, as well as parallel bars, benches, and high rings. The athletes who came to perform were muscled and fit but nothing like the hulking weight lifters of the York Gang. Agility and balance were prized as much as strength. Plus there were women.

There was Paula Unger Boelsems, a crowd favorite with an eye-popping figure, who did daring athletic flips and was strong enough, even at 110 pounds, to tear telephone books in half for a Movietone newsreel. There was Relna Brewer, sister of stuntman Paul Brewer, who lifted weights and tossed men in the air. There was the stunning Beverly Jocher who could balance 590 pounds of men on her tiny frame — and went on to become Miss Southern California and Miss Pacific Coast.

Most famous of all was Abbye "Pudgy" Stockton, an icon of Muscle Beach and a pivotal figure in the history of women's exercise. Before Stockton, the few women who trained with weights were professional strongwomen, Amazonian bulked-up lifters who confirmed a common shibboleth — that weights robbed a woman of feminine sex appeal. Stockton put that myth to rest.

"At the end of the depression," wrote Jan Todd, in a eulogy to Stockton, "petite Pudgy Stockton with her glowing skin, shining hair, miraculous curves and amazing strength appeared on the golden sands of Muscle Beach and became emblematic of the new type of woman America needed to win the War. Competent, feminine, strong, yet sexy, Pudgy made America's young men pant with desire, and also pant in their gyms as they tried to prove themselves worthy of her."

She grew up in Santa Monica, a solid if chunky teenager (hence the nickname, courtesy of her father) who went to work as a telephone operator after high school, a sedentary job that saw her weight shoot up to 140. Her boyfriend, Les Stockton, a student and athlete at the University of California, Los Angeles (UCLA), suggested weights as a way of reducing and bought her a York training course. Trimmed down, she finally worked up the nerve to appear on the beach in a makeshift two-piece bathing suit, which her mother had designed by ripping apart an old brassiere. She was an instant sensation. She supported husband-to-be

Les, who weighed 180 pounds, in an overhead handstand; she hoisted weights and did complicated gymnastic feats or flew through the air to land in her fiancé's arms. The photographers came running. In 1939 Pudgy was featured in *Look*, *Pic*, and Macfadden's *Physical Culture*. She appeared in the newsreels *Whatta Build* and *Muscle Town USA*. By the end of the 1940s, her body would grace forty-two magazine covers from around the world and she had begun a regular column for *Strength and Health* called "Barbelles."

The outbreak of World War II took a toll on the fun in the sand at Muscle Beach, as it did everywhere. Men were suddenly in short supply. However, the war also worked to drive a new enthusiasm for fitness. The armed forces needed recruits in shape who could fight. Some who had gotten a taste for bodybuilding carried that passion into conflict. George Eiferman, a skinny, bullied boy from Philadelphia, had gotten a taste for bodybuilding from the York Gang. When war broke out, he took his weights onto a navy ship and emerged at war's end with a muscle-packed body and dreams of becoming Mr. America. In thrall with Muscle Beach, he eventually made the cross-country trek and landed a trainer's job at one of the nascent gyms started by Santa Monica regular Vic Tanny. Known as "Genial George" thanks to a fun sense of humor, Eiferman was one of the beach's best-loved musclemen whose signature stunt was to lift a 135-pound barbell with his left hand while he played the "Hawaiian War Chant" on his trumpet. He won the Amateur Athletic Union's (AAU) 1948 Mr. America crown, devoted years to touring schools and inspiring youth, then returned to competitive bodybuilding after a twelve-year layoff and was awarded the "Professional Mr. Universe" title in 1962.

Few were as popular as Eiferman, few Muscle Beach standouts even became household names, but many fashioned highly successful careers. Show business was an obvious choice, with many going on to bit parts in Hollywood and stunt work. Russ Saunders, lanky and handsome, would become a contract stuntman for Warner Brothers and doubled in films for Douglas Fairbanks and Gene Kelly. His own star turn came the day he got a surprise call from Warner Bros. boss Jack Warner, who summoned him to his office to meet none other than Salvador Dalí. The artist was scouring Hollywood for a model for Jesus in his painting *Christ of St. John of the Cross*. Up until his death the license plate on Saunders's modest Toyota read "DALI2."

The most famous movie alum of Muscle Beach was Steve Reeves. The son of a Montana farmer, who died in a harvesting accident, he moved with his family to Oakland and got into serious training with Ed Yarick at Yarick's Physical Culture Studio. He did a nineteen-month stint in the Philippines, where awestruck villagers called him the "White God." The war over, he made the pilgrimage to Santa Monica, roomed with George Eiferman, and created a major stir on the beach, thanks to his sensational build and chiseled good looks.

"You'd know him a mile away by the incredible V-shaped torso, tapering from wide shoulders down to a tiny wasp waist," remembered Joe Weider, who first spotted Reeves on Muscle Beach, where Weider also hung out. "Up close, you saw the handsomest bodybuilder of all time, hands down. . . . I'll never forget the mobs of people stopping and staring when he and I walked up Broadway. He wasn't a celebrity yet, but he absolutely dazzled them. Steve mesmerized women. With him around, other guys felt invisible."

As a bodybuilder, Reeves reached his peak with the 1948 "Mr. World" title in Cannes, then lost a celebrated "Mr. Universe" showdown in London to John Grimek. His acting talent, unfortunately, never matched his looks or muscles. He had only two speaking roles — in the musical *Athena*, as a pal of Jane Powell's character, and in the Ed Wood film *Jail Bait*, playing a cop — before his career was rescued by a series of low-budget Italian sword-and-sandal epics. He played Hercules twice — in *Hercules* and *Hercules Unchained* — then starred in a half-dozen other films as bare-chested Greek, Tatar, and Malaysian warriors. After the box-office smash of *Hercules*, he turned down the role that finally went to Clint Eastwood in Sergio Leone's *A Fistful of Dollars*, refusing to believe that "Italians could make a western." All his parts were dubbed. He did most of his own stunts, however, which contributed to an early retirement: filming *The Last Days of Pompeii*, he injured his shoulder when his chariot slammed into a tree.

Throughout the 1940s and into the 1950s, Muscle Beach retained its reputation as the prime showplace for tanned athletes and extravagant muscle. Even Hollywood bombshells dropped by to enjoy the spectacle; Jayne Mansfield, who eventually married bodybuilder Mickey Hargitay, was a frequent visitor, along with Jane Russell, who was pursuing Bob Waterfield, the football star she ended up marrying. Babe Didrikson, the great track and field star, put in time on the beach, as did Olympic skater and actress Sonja Henie.

And then there was Mae West. Her film career as the naughty sexpot had long since stuttered to a close when, in 1954, at age sixty-two, she decided to reinvent herself with a nightclub act. It was Eiferman who obliged her call for beefcake by recruiting a group of his Muscle Beach pals to audition in her Hollywood apartment. West cast half a dozen and launched a nationwide tour, opening at the Sahara in Las Vegas. The highlight had West lounging provocatively on a sofa as the men strode out, backs to the audience, then, to West's delight, parting their robes. Later they strutted their stuff in tiny toga-style briefs and sandals. The revue proved a huge hit, playing to sellout crowds, a ribald finale to West's career.

If the legacy of Muscle Beach were just about Mr. Universe titles and men in skimpy briefs, it might not remain such a benchmark in the history of fitness. In fact, it served another purpose. It was where the modern gym began.

There had been gyms before, most famously the singular Manhattan studio of lightweight Prussian strongman Sigmund "Sig" Klein. Klein had come to New York in 1924 to consult with Professor Attila, the legendary mentor of Sandow, only to find Attila had just died. In short order he married Attila's daughter and took over his gym, then moved it to the heart of the theater district, where it became a magnet for Broadway's biggest names and home to an extraordinary collection of muscleman photos and artifacts. Away from the glitter of Broadway, however, even in sunny California, most gyms were dingy basement hangouts stocked with basic weights or crude makeshift devices. High school and college workout rooms, rarely with better equipment, were for football players and wrestlers. "Even then," noted journalist Marla Matzer Rose, "[they] were kept under lock and key; too dangerous not to mention unnatural for anyone to get near. Many coaches banned weight training entirely."

The gym at Muscle Beach was worse than most. It sat beneath a decrepit five-story hotel and was affectionately known as "the Dungeon." The equipment was enough to scare anyone: milk crates and splintered plywood for benches and racks, dumbbells that rattled at broken welds, pulleys and cable salvaged from a nearby boatyard. Few have described it more vividly than Dave Draper, a gym regular and future Mr. Universe: "Two long steep staircases penetrated the eternal dimness, illumination coming from three strategically located 60-watt bulbs. The concrete floor was cracked and bulging, the walls crumbling and ceiling 12 feet overhead was sagging, especially where the ground floor bar leaked beerlike brownish ooze. An ankle-deep puddle formed near the squat rack each winter and nobody used the shower or toilet except in emergencies." It was, noted Draper with more loyalty than irony, "unquestionably the greatest gym in the world."

GYMS GET A FACELIFT

The idea of opening a gym was a tempting option for regulars at Muscle Beach, both to spread the gospel and to launch a moneymaking career. It was not easy. Then, as now, the gym and health club business was a daunting challenge that required equal parts capital, service expertise, and sales savvy. Eiferman was among the musclemen who tried a few, shut them, and left it at that. More successful was Pudgy Stockton, who capitalized on her appeal to women with her Salon of Figure Development, "Specializing in Bust Development, Figure Contouring, Reducing," read a promotional postcard. She started on Sunset Boulevard, then opened branches in the more affluent communities of Beverly Hills and Pasadena. In both locations her husband, Les, opened a men's gym next door.

Few of these gyms delivered a solid clientele or guaranteed income. Most were limited to bodybuilders, the restless housewife (in Pudgy's case), and a smattering of movie stars. What was needed was a new marketing concept and, just possibly, a new type of gym. It might have evolved naturally. Instead, like so much else in the history of fitness, it sprang full-blown from an entrepreneurial visionary, though there is some dispute as to who deserves that "visionary" title. Jack LaLanne long claimed to have invented the modern health club, but his first club opened in Oakland in 1936. Across the continent, in the unlikely city of Rochester, New York, another club opened in 1935. Its founder would soon make the pilgrimage to Muscle Beach. But back then he was a full-time schoolteacher, the son of a tailor, who opened the gym in his parents' garage. It featured bright colors, carpeting, and background music. His name was Vic Tanny.

There were, in fact, two Tannys—Vic and his younger brother

Armand. Of the two Armand was the more strapping hunk and would place fifth in the great 1949 "Professional Mr. USA" contest, an unprecedented show of glamour and muscle that featured Grimek (the winner) along with Reeves and Eiferman. Armand had planned on becoming a doctor and headed west in 1939 to pursue his medical degree at the University of Southern California, though his passion had already turned to weight lifting. He was soon joined by brother Vic with an equally lukewarm plot to advance his education (he was there for a teacher's degree). Spurred by Vic's ambition, the brothers emptied their five-hundred-dollar joint bank account, borrowed another two hundred dollars, and opened the first West Coast Tanny gym in a second-story loft near the Santa Monica Beach in 1939. In 1941 they added two more — one in the tony shopping district on Wilshire Boulevard, another in Long Beach. The latter quickly shut after Pearl Harbor and the coastal blackouts that followed; the other succumbed to the surge of men heading off to fight. But the end of the war saw Tanny back with a vengeance. His new location was a seven-thousand-square-foot former USO facility in Santa Monica, and it soon became the hub of every famous Muscle Beach regular, including Reeves, Eiferman, and future gym heavyweight Joe Gold.

That was just the beginning. Tanny had gotten a taste for business — big business. "His equation was a simple one," noted Rose. "More gyms equaled more people equaled more money." It was a time when branded retail and restaurant chains were beginning to spread in America, and Tanny thought, why not fitness shops? "Shops" were not at all what he had in mind, however. His dream was to rescue the gym from its grungy reputation and turn it into a welcoming palace that would lure middle-class strivers with lavish surroundings and bright, new equipment. With that prescription in mind, he began opening clubs throughout Southern California, then spread the franchise across North America. In a matter of years, he had an eighty-four-club empire that grossed an annual fifteen million dollars.

The club motto was, "Take it off, build it up, and make it firm." But there were plenty of other reasons to pay membership dues. Some clubs had bowling alleys with what was then a major innovation — automatic pin setters; many had movie screens and ballet classes. There were ice skating rinks in Tyrolean settings with Swiss chalets and ice dyed pink. Passersby could be treated to the sight of swaying palm trees through immense plate-glass windows, a precursor of many a modern health club with its sweating treadmill runner on full display. But Tanny's clubs were less about flaunting the hard-core exerciser than in satisfying an upwardly mobile clientele craving a place to kick back and revel in the promise of the Eisenhower fifties. The pitch was less perspiration than aspiration, and Tanny was anointed the era's dream maker. A hard-cover magazine of the time, *Wisdom*, placed him on its December 1961 cover, following issues that featured Albert Einstein, Walt Disney, and Jesus, and had this to say of its newest icon:

> Entering a Tanny Health Center is like walking into a glittering wonderland. Underfoot, one feels the deep, soft pile of the rich red carpets; subdued indirect lighting casts a warm rosy glow all about and the strains of muted music fall lightly and soothingly on the ear. In these relaxed exquisite surroundings, people of all age groups are busily engaged in acquiring better figures and more abundant, vibrant health. . . . The sparkling swimming pools, with exotic South Sea murals decorating the walls on every side, the inviting lounge chairs and umbrellas on the pool decks, give one the impression of being in an exclusive country club.

Tanny clearly got carried away with his own vision. His extravagance knew no bounds; one of his most opulent endeavors was a gilded gym that was completely finished in gold plating, down to the barbells and dumbbells. The excesses were the occasional source of merry parody, in part thanks to Tanny's name. In the movie *Muscle Beach Party*, Don Rickles played a trainer named "Jack Fanny"; he was immortalized in *Mad Magazine*'s "Vic Tinny" issue. In the 1963 movie *The Nutty Professor*, starring Jerry Lewis, the gym itself got the wacko treatment.

Not all, however, was a laughing matter. In addition to his upscale makeover, Tanny pioneered another innovation: annual memberships. The haphazard pay-as-you-go strategy had done little to build reliable capital for maintenance or expansion. Tanny might have promised a country-club haven, but his methods of signing up members were street tough. "Volume is what counts," he proclaimed in a 1961 *Time* article, which also cited an internal daily memo that went out to sales staff: "If you fail to get an appointment, then take a gun out of the desk and shoot yourself." Salesmen were expected to put pressure on prospects to join, intimidating them as necessary; each day's top seller was rewarded by becoming the next day's sales manager. There were so many complaints from Vic Tanny members and customers that the New York State attorney general forced all gyms to sign a fair-practices code that prohibited methods of selling that were deceitful, misleading, or fraudulent. The constraints put a crimp on business, which bore resemblance to a Ponzi scheme: sign up as many members as possible in one location, and then use that anticipated revenue stream as collateral to borrow the money to open the next gym.

The downfall was quick. Behind in payments and taxes, the business falling on hard times, Tanny unloaded many of his clubs to new owners and "retired" to Florida, where his few attempts at restoring his name and the brand went nowhere. He died there in 1985 at the age of seventy-three after suffering a debilitating stroke.

Armand escaped this ignominious end. He managed the company in its fifties heyday, took a leave to join Mae West's nightclub act, and then became a features editor for the magazine *Muscle and Fitness*, published by Joe Weider. He kept up an active lifestyle – weight training, running, and cycling – and maintained a strict raw-food diet, a habit he had picked up in a postwar visit to Samoa, where he was impressed by the stalwart natives. He turned off his stove for good in 1948 and lived another sixty-one years, dying of natural causes in 2009 at age ninety.

Muscle Beach itself died its own natural death, though there were contributing factors. The notion of a robust masculinity so flagrantly displayed on the sunny sands had come to seem limited, if not suspect. Men who shaved their bodies and posed in tiny tight trunks no longer seemed quite so iconic in a sexually liberated culture. There were hints of homosexuality and the occasional charge of promiscuity. Even the editors of *Strength and Health*, Hoffman's magazine, saw fit to comment on the sordid gossip in a 1957 issue: "Rumors may have reached you that some queer proceedings transpired on the Beach. We have heard of some pretty odd goings-on ourselves, but we never actually caught anybody in flagrant delicto (or whatever the legal phrase is) on one of our personal visits. Naturally a lot of guys and gals pitch a bit of woo – this is standard procedure on any beach."

The following year a sex scandal involving several men – two of them York weight lifters – and a couple of underage girls was enough for the city of Santa Monica. It dismantled the equipment and platforms and bulldozed the sand, turning most of the famed playground into a parking lot. A few years later the scene migrated two miles south to Venice Beach. Though that location would generate its own fame, thanks to a new generation of bodybuilders and gym entrepreneurs, the original Muscle Beach was where it all started, the home to alumni that included not just Tanny but the other claimant to the title "Father of the Modern Health Club," the one and only Jack LaLanne.

JACK LALANNE WORKS "THE BACK PORCH"

By his own reckoning, LaLanne did not grow up with prospects of becoming a legend. It seemed questionable that he would survive adolescence. "At 15 I knew the tortures of the damned," he liked to lament. "I was a sick shut-in! I wouldn't go out and see people. I had pimples, boils, flat feet, bad eyes, bony arms and legs and my overall disposition was rotten to the core. I lived on sugar. I was a sugarholic. I was so weak I couldn't participate in sports. I didn't want anyone to see me."

Born in 1914 to French immigrant parents in San Francisco, he was in such poor condition that he dropped out of school for a year and might have dropped out of life permanently had his mother not dragged him to a Paul Bragg nutrition crusade. Bragg was a big name at the time, an apostle of Bernarr Macfadden and a health food evangelist. Not all of Bragg's later claims to immortality stand up to scrutiny—first to open a health food store, first to introduce pineapple and tomato juices to America, first to import a hand juicer. But he was tireless in his promotion of better health through nutrition, both on his daily radio health programs and on his cross-country tours. The list of people whose lives he claimed to have changed ranged from J. C. Penney, Dr. Scholl, and Conrad Hilton to Olympic gold medalists, including his cousin Dan Bragg, the pole-vaulting star. Of them all, LaLanne would become his most popular success.

Spotting LaLanne about to exit his event, he waved him forward and got LaLanne to confess his diet of cakes, pies, and ice cream, whereupon Bragg, a rabid vegetarian, called him "a walking garbage can." Shamed into swearing off sugar, LaLanne took Bragg's advice and began his miraculous turnaround. He stopped eating sweets and meat (at least temporarily; Armand Tanny recalled visiting a local stockyard with

LaLanne to acquire cow's blood to drink when LaLanne was in training). He began lifting weights at the Berkeley YMCA; he read everything he could get his hands on about fitness and the body, including *Gray's Anatomy*; he studied premed and graduated from a chiropractic college. Imbued with a mission to help others get in shape, he opened his pioneering gym in Oakland in 1936. He worked there fourteen hours a day and then hopped in his car and drove four hundred miles through the night for the morning fun at Muscle Beach.

He was far from the biggest stud on the sand. A mere five-foot-four, he developed a serious chest but got much more mileage from his effervescent personality and folksy manner—the ideal mix for the new medium of television. He started his first show in 1951 after a stint in the South Pacific during World War II and a hitch teaching calisthenics in the navy. Dressed in a skin-hugging jumper and black ballet slippers, he led a thirty-minute exercise class as if he were standing ten feet away on the living-room floor. The immediacy was a breakthrough for television itself, a nonstop personal chat that mixed jokes, anatomy tips, recipes, product pitches, and, of course, his own brand of calisthenics. "One and a two and a three and four," he would chant as he lifted his knee, then dropped to the floor for push-ups. "You know, students, exercise makes you feel real good all over, doesn't it? Do you know why? It's because it makes the blood race through your body and because it massages your internal organs. But now, let's get back to Trimnastics—you, too, Cuddles and Francine, on your feet—and go to work on the back porch."

He worked with an offstage organ player and a dog, Happy, who alternately slouched half-asleep on a rug at the back of the set or trotted up with a note announcing, "It's Glamour Stretch Time!" The Glamour Stretcher, essentially an elastic rope, was the top product LaLanne pushed on air, selling upwards of forty thousand a month. He marketed vitamins—"delicious" wild-cherry protein wafers, a face lotion "to keep skin glowingly moist," and a "high-fashion silhouette blue exercise suit, ideal, too, for marketing and gardening." He also sold the Jack LaLanne Face Exerciser—a rubber device that was inserted into the mouth for muscle flexing. All told, his business grossed three million dollars in 1960.

The show was a huge hit. In Los Angeles, where it originated, the show pulled almost as many viewers as the six other television stations combined. Its success turned LaLanne into the darling of journalists who loved to report on his antic personality and what *Newsweek* termed his "remarkable mix of wheat germ and cornball," even as they tried to fathom his appeal. "What LaLanne was selling was a sort of fundamental religion that he devoutly believed in—and still does," ventured one writer. "He was simply a physical culturist, like Charles Atlas or Vic Tanny, but he had the congregation and they didn't."

He also had a canny partner. In 1958 he met Henry C. Akerberg, a longtime vice president of Macmillan Petroleum Corporation, who left Macmillan after thirty years to form LaLanne, Inc. ("The House That Health Built"), and went about turning the company into a marketing powerhouse. Akerberg played a key role in promoting the television show, which was soon accessible to 50 percent of the U.S. population, and plotted expansion into South America, England, and Australia, "wherever the family of man can be benefited," he said, and added, "The way things are going, we can almost see Jack as a world power."

Akerberg was also a businessman with a shrewd sense of product image. He directed that LaLanne's "Desiccated Liver Tablets" be renamed "Liver, Iron, and Vitamin B-12 Tablets," and he shut down manufacture of the Face Exerciser, which required users to clamp it in their teeth and tug. "Too many of our students," he explained, "wore dentures."

When LaLanne was not encouraging the housewives of America to work on their "back porch," he was luring them into clubs. LaLanne was a lot more practical than Tanny. He cared about growing his franchise—at the peak his name would be associated with more than two hundred clubs—but he also wanted to improve the environment of exercise. He was unique in his appeal to women, whom he urged to work out with weights. His biggest female fan was his blonde wife, Elaine, who ran his office and did all his exercise routines, adding pounds to her once-thin frame and three inches to her bust. "Man, she has a terrific body," LaLanne liked to boast. "What I've done is to build her to my own specifications."

He wrote books. He put out tapes and DVDs; *Hydronastics* was a "water and exercise" video, and *Face-A-Tronics* was "designed for the facial and neck muscles." He sold anything and everything—vitamins, supplements, assorted workout devices, and, of course, the juicer. As a public speaker and media personality, he immortalized dozens of "LaLanne-isms" that included "Your waistline is your lifeline," "Better to wear out than rust out," and "Do — don't stew." He had a standing challenge for anyone to match his morning walk. He like to boast that he held the world record for push-ups, once pumping out one thousand in twenty-four minutes. His most celebrated stunt was towing a one-thousand-ton boat through the treacherous waters between Alcatraz and Fisherman's Wharf in San Francisco — handcuffed and shackled.

In the wash of history, LaLanne's celebrity and brand empire tend to obscure the fact that he was not alone in promoting the habit of healthy eating and exercise. He was not even the first on network television. That honor belongs to a woman who, long before Jane Fonda instilled a passion for Lycra among millions of housewives, was billed as "the First Lady of Fitness Fashion." More significantly, she roused fifties America from what many, including the man in the White House, regarded as a dangerous torpor.

BONNIE PRUDDEN SHOCKS THE PRESIDENT

The mid-1950s were marked by a serious case of Cold War jitters. The Soviet Union was flexing its nuclear muscle and, in 1957, would launch *Sputnik*, sparking a national anxiety that the Communists would soon dominate space. The Korean War had done little to assure Americans that their way of life would prevail. Retreat from the Korean peninsula and the failure to achieve a decisive victory left many looking for scapegoats, and much of the blame was laid to domestic weakness. It did not help that when the United States and the Soviet Union did confront one another, face-to-face, the Americans suffered a crushing defeat. The Soviets dominated the 1952 Olympic Games at Helsinki, and only a last-day bounty of boxing gold medals allowed the Americans to salvage a measure of pride. Four years later, in the Cortina d'Ampezzo Winter Games, the Soviets demolished the United States in total team scores.

The Olympics fiasco confirmed what had been a brewing concern at home. Americans were out of shape. This fear was underscored as the country again sent its fighting men abroad to war. Between the Selective Service inception in 1948 and on through the fifties, up until Kennedy's inauguration in 1961, 39 percent of the six million registrants given preinduction examinations were rejected for either physical, mental, or emotional reasons. The most disturbing evidence came in 1955 with a devastating report on youth fitness, which found that Americans fell way behind their counterparts in Europe. With a sample of seventy-five hundred participants, U.S. youngsters flunked a battery of minimal tests that included sit-ups, leg lifts, and toe touches.

The evidence had first appeared in the *New York State Journal of Medicine* and caught the attention of John Kelly, a Philadelphia financier and national sculling champion, though also known as the father of actress Grace Kelly. Horrified, Kelly passed the report on to Pennsylvania senator James Duff, who immediately convened a White House luncheon with President Dwight D. Eisenhower. The luncheon was a high-profile meeting of White House executives and what *Sports Illustrated* called "the greatest array of U.S. sports stars ever gathered together in one place"—thirty athletes that included Willie Mays, Bob Cousy, Tony Trabert, Bill Russell, Hank Greenberg, and Archie Moore, as well as baseball commissioner Ford Frick. Less recognizable was one of only two women in the room, a trim, lively brunette who had coauthored the report, though she, too, was a serious athlete. A world-class mountain climber, she had become a legend on the towering rocks of upstate New York's Shawangunk range, otherwise known as "the Gunks." The woman had put up a record thirty "first ascents" on the Gunks, climbs that bore names including "the Brat" and "Bonnie's Roof." Her full name was Bonnie Prudden.

Born in 1914 in Manhattan, the same year as LaLanne, she had evinced her fearless love of climbing early. As a four-year-old, she had terrified her parents by squeezing out her second-floor nursery window, then traversing a six-inch ledge and shimmying down a tree to wander the neighboring streets at night. At the suggestion of doctors, who recommended discipline and physical exhaustion, she was enrolled in rigorous ballet classes, which not only cured her daredevil wandering but also launched her brief career as a professional dancer (she appeared on Broadway in *Life Begins at 8:40*, starring Bert Lahr and Ray Bolger). In her early twenties she had switched to skiing and mountain climbing and became one of the top female climbers in the world. On her honeymoon she and her husband, a wealthy manufacturer, climbed the Matterhorn. When she suffered a traumatic pelvis fracture in a skiing accident, she was told her she would never be able to climb or ski again, let alone have children. She was in traction for five months. Within a few years she had two daughters and, in 1943, earned a National Ski Patrol badge, the first ever awarded a woman.

Her lifetime interest in physical education was cemented the day she went to check on her eight-year-old daughter's required forty-minute exercise class at a public school. "I was horrified," she later recalled. "The first ten minutes of the class were spent calling attendance, then another ten minutes dismissing students with illegitimate excuses. The teacher wore a skirt and high heels and a whistle around her neck as 25 little girls played circles games for 20 minutes."

She promptly began teaching classes of her own, gathering her daughters—her second child was then four—and recruiting five friends of each. "At first, two mothers called me to say that they didn't want their daughters to exercise because they would 'get muscles.' I told them, 'Under every curve is a muscle. No muscles, no curves.'"

She soon had seventy-five kids, changed the name of the class from "Exercise" to "Conditioning," got schools to lend her their gyms, and had enrollment jump to two hundred weekly. Outside of class, everywhere else she looked, the children seemed badly out of shape, a condition she ascribed to a nation of "couch potatoism, [to] school buses, cars and television." At the time, she and her husband frequently climbed with a man named Hans Kraus, a professor of physical rehabilitation at Columbia Presbyterian Hospital and the cocreator of a fitness test with a physician named Sonya Weber. The test measured basic strength and flexibility, including sit-ups, leg lifts, and toe touches. Prudden was climbing one day with Kraus, "resting on a ledge thousands of feet up in the mountains," when she asked if there were not some way to document her kids' improvement over a year. He gave her the Kraus-Weber Test.

The results dismayed both Kraus and Prudden. More than 50 percent of her incoming students failed the test. More concerned than ever, Prudden began testing more and more children. Wherever she and Kraus climbed—Austria, Italy, Switzerland—she took time to contact local schools and administer the test. She took side trips to India and South America and tested children there. She grew even more appalled at what she was finding. The Europeans and non-American children did fine, failing less than 10 percent of the tests; children in the United States scored an average 40 percent failure rate. Together, Prudden and Kraus began writing papers to publicize what they had found.

She was understandably nervous to find herself at the White House luncheon, but when Eisenhower gave her an encouraging smile she relaxed and talked him through the report. She demonstrated the simple exercises and said of the failure of so many young Americans to pass, "Can you imagine?" Eisenhower shook his head and replied, "I'm shocked."

Prudden's testimony quickly became known as "the report that shocked the president." Eisenhower was sufficiently disturbed that he directed Vice President Richard Nixon to immediately set up a conference and take action. Within months Eisenhower signed off on the historic cabinet-level President's Council on the Fitness of Youth.

The report she had coauthored had a profound impact on physical education and did much to spur attention to fitness. In the tense atmosphere of the Cold War, it was a rallying cry to reassess the debilitated body and even the national character. The executive director of Eisenhower's council, Shane McCarthy, saw fit to address the question of "What's wrong with youth?" by denouncing "a culture which is prone to substitute license for freedom, hedonism for liberty, irresponsibility for obligation, inertia for challenge and over-programming for opportunity. The subject of youth fitness is a most important ingredient not only for our strength but also for our survival."

McCarthy was not alone in his flourishes of rhetoric, or in the abiding anxiety that America, and especially its youth, had gone flabby. An article in the Parent-Teacher Association magazine threw out the troubling headline "Is Youth Lost in the Wilds of the Suburbs?" and went on to excoriate a complacent nation in which adolescents fell victim to conformism and lost their moral compass.

That same lament for a weakened backbone continued through the fifties. In an article that appeared six days after the 1957 launch of *Sputnik*, Walter Lippmann claimed that America had floundered under the "enormous fallacy that the highest purpose of the American social order is to multiply the enjoyment of consumer goods" and urged Americans to reassess priorities, to "look inward upon ourselves and concern ourselves with our own failings, and be determined not so much to beat the Russians as to cure ourselves."

President John F. Kennedy's inaugural exhortation—"Ask not what your country can do for you—ask what you can do for your country" — was the natural extension of this call to embrace a new rigor. Just three weeks before, in a December 1960 *Sports Illustrated* article he authored, "The Soft American," he had linked youth fitness to Cold War foreign policy. "In a very real and immediate sense," he wrote, "our growing softness, our increasing lack of physical fitness, is a menace to our national security." Much as World War II had been won on the playing fields of Eton, "the stamina and strength which the defense of liberty requires are not the product of a few weeks' basic training or a month's conditioning. These only come from bodies which have been conditioned by a lifetime of participation in sports and interest in physical activity. Our struggles against aggressors throughout our history have been won on the playgrounds and corner lots and fields of America."

Prudden was gratified to have brought the fitness crisis to the national stage, but she remained frustrated by the lack of progress. Not enough was being done, she complained. It was not a charge that applied to Prudden. She expanded the Institute for Physical Fitness she had opened in White Plains, New York, and helped condition thousands of people — "young girls and boys, athletes, Westchester matrons and gents as well as Olympic ski teams." One of her athletes, Penny Pitou, took a silver medal in the Olympics. In 1956 her book *Is Your Child Really Fit?* was published by Harper & Row. When the so-called Space Age began in 1957 with the launch of *Sputnik*, she put out FITNIK: *The Bonnie Prudden Fitness Test Kit.* She was forty-three the year she presented her report to Eisenhower; the following year she appeared on the cover of *Sports Illustrated*, the first female athlete to do so, in an issue that announced "a nationwide report on physical fitness" and, in even bigger, bolder type, heralded Prudden in a new series of "illustrated lessons on how to keep fit." The photo displayed her in a sky-blue leotard emblazoned with tiny stars, her body twisted in upside-down contortion, face pressed sideways against the floor, beaming encouragement.

Within months she was invited by Arlene Francis and Hugh Downs to host a weekly exercise segment on CBS's *Home Show*. ("Leotards and tights were signals to exercise," she later explained at the launch of her Fitness Fashion line of exercise wear.) She soon switched to the even larger audience that watched *The Today Show* on NBC and followed that with her own syndicated fitness show in the 1960s. As promised she wrote dozens of fitness columns for *Sports Illustrated* and went on to author fifteen books. She devised some of the first fitness classes for infants, toddlers, even the blind, and set up hundreds of exercise programs in schools, hospitals, camps, factories, prisons, and mental institutions. She pioneered mother-baby swim classes for infants. She invented exercise equipment and one of the first climbing walls.

Few people, men or women, ever equaled the contributions she made to fitness.

CHAPTER 4

The Machine Age, 1960s–1970s

Arthur Jones invents the Nautilus; Ray Wilson and Augie Nieto launch the Lifecycle; the dance world comes knocking at Joe Pilates's door

THE WILD KINGDOM OF ARTHUR JONES

Building muscle took work. For the better part of civilized history, most everyone relied on the barbell or dumbbell. Improvements happened slowly. In 1902 Alan Calvert founded the Milo Barbell Company—the first to mass-produce weights. Previously, weight lifters had to vary the weights by filling the globes with shot or sand. Calvert came up with the idea of plate-loaded barbells; to adjust the resistance you simply clapped on more iron. Calvert had first gotten interested in weight lifting after spotting Sandow at the 1893 Chicago World's Fair and would go on to write the classic 1924 book on weight training, *Super Strength*. He scorned the nutritionists of his time, believing that exercise stimulated the proper appetite for food—and drink. To prove his point, he cited the heavyweight champ John L. Sullivan, who once won a bet by downing one hundred mixed drinks in a single evening.

Machines, such as they were, were mostly faddist oddities or highly specialized. Windship, the Harvard physician, had a device that used air pressure to vary resistance. It was not until Muscle Beach that the culture of bigger, better muscles led to more enduring inventions. It was Jack LaLanne who invented the leg-extension machine, then contrived a piece of equipment that enabled users to lift heavy weights on guided rails; it was improved and popularized by a Vic Tanny employee, Rudy Smith, and became known as the Smith machine. Harold Zinkin, a Muscle Beach regular and 1941 Mr. California winner, designed the first pin-loaded weight stack, then expanded his idea to create the multistation Universal Machine. Safer than hefting dumbbells or barbells, it also obviated the need to thump around the gym floor and, in time, proved an efficient way to run a school team, say, through a workout. In 1964 it was selling a unit a week and would expand, after Zinkin sold the company, to slap its brand on a broad array of fitness equipment, from benches to bikes and treadmills.

But a true breakthrough in technology had yet to occur. That situation was about to change with two machines that would revolutionize the habit of exercise. Though utterly different in makeup and purpose, the machines would soon dominate the industry, each the basis for giants in manufacture and sales.

Like their machines, the men who launched them were not soon forgotten. Born within a year of each other, in 1912 and 1913, Arthur Jones and Ray Wilson were both rough men, combative, tough to get along with. Neither had anything like a formal education. Jones barely made it to high school; Wilson dropped out in tenth grade. Whoever met them or did business with one rarely came away unchanged by the experience. Each liked to get his way; each brought a measure of bullheaded swagger to his work. They were not men you wanted to cross.

It was 1974 when Wilson first heard of Jones—and from him. He was in his California office, where he presided over the group of clubs called Family Fitness, the latest of his club chains that included American Health Studios, Silhouette, and European Health Spas. He was used to sweet talk from suppliers peddling merchandise to put in his clubs. The man on the phone did not waste time with sweet talk.

"I'm Arthur Jones," he said. "Have you heard of me? I invented equipment that's going to replace all equipment in gyms."

"Okay, I'll try a line of it," Wilson agreed.

"You don't understand English very well, do you?" said Jones. "I said, it's replacing *all* equipment."

The equipment was Nautilus, named after the scalloped shell, and was designed to make lifting weights simpler. Instead of juggling plates, bars, and bolts, a user had simply to shift a pin in the machine's weight stack. Better yet, unlike other machines of the time, it employed a system of pulleys and cams to ensure constant resistance on a lifter's muscles during the entire range of motion. It made exercise both easier and more efficient.

Jones had unveiled his first machine at a weight-lifting convention in Los Angeles in 1970, having hauled it there cross-country in a trailer from his home in Florida. A perfectionist, he constantly tinkered with the design. When the modification did not work or the machine was deemed less than perfect, Jones made sure none of his competitors—if there were any—would steal his work. He dug a huge hole with his bulldozer and buried it in the ground. The machine graveyard made a significant impression on Wilson when Jones first invited him to his ranch in Florida, ten years after that first phone conversation. "Arthur was a genius—I'm no fucking genius," said Wilson. "I don't know anything about equipment, I just know how to push people around. But what Arthur did was amazing. His whole operation there was as crazy as he was. It was so far beyond business—it had nothing to do with anything but Arthur."

The "whole operation," as Wilson puts it, was called Jumbolair, a two-hundred-acre ranch on the outskirts of Gainesville. By the time of Wilson's visit, it had become a tourist site. There was a private zoo, filled with snakes and giant crocodiles. Jones had a hospital and rehab clinic staffed by doctors who treated injured pro football players, many from the Miami Dolphins. There was the airstrip, big enough to land his Boeing 707; other planes were flown by Jones's teenage wife, whom he had sent to pilot school to learn to fly. There was Jones himself, a profane, tough-talking chain-smoker who swilled quarts of coffee each day and strode around in horn-rimmed glasses and ill-fitting corduroys with a holstered Colt .45.

That first visit between the men went well for a while. They were two rough diamonds, each passionate about his work, each committed to revolutionizing the fitness landscape. But after several days the hospitality wore thin, and Jones, fueled by increasing amounts of wine, turned belligerent and threatened to beat Wilson up. Wilson, muscled and wiry, had once been an amateur wrestler, fighting in 104 bouts and never losing. "I told him it wouldn't be a matter of beating," said Wilson. "It would be who would kill the other guy first."

The belligerence was likely owed less to wine than to Jones's combative nature—and his contempt for competition. Wilson was then a millionaire many times over, having secured rights to a piece of equipment called the Lifecycle. It had taken him five years to develop the machine and have it installed in the clubs he ran. Jones, the inventor of Nautilus, was not a big fan of people running nowhere on treadmill-like devices to pump up their heart rate. He had little respect for Dr. Kenneth Cooper, who had promoted the field of cardiofitness. "Aerobic exercises," Jones told an interviewer, were "worthless for any purpose"; in the same interview he called Cooper "a borderline idiot who knows nothing about constructive exercise."

Wilson ended that first visit early. He went back to Jumbolair twice, each time ducking out after a day or two, claiming he had other business. Wilson was no one to back away from a fight, but he had his limits. As a man who knew Jones well put it: "Arthur could be downright dangerous."

Jones was born into an upper-middle-class family of doctors in small-town Arkansas in 1926. When he was in his early teens, the family moved to the rowdy oil boomtown of Seminole, Oklahoma, to set up a new medical practice. Seminole, Jones would later write, was filled with "whores, gunfighters, thieves and general riff-raff of every sort. The jail could not hold them so they were chained like animals to pieces of pipe driven into the ground. Anyone with any common sense carried a gun." Jones's father owned a double-barreled ten-gauge shotgun pistol; Jones himself had the permit for a concealed pistol. He dropped out of school in ninth grade ("I should have dropped out in sixth grade") and began a vagabond childhood, running away from home to hitchhike, jump freight trains, or sneak passage on tramp steamers. A self-proclaimed prodigy, he claimed to have read his father's entire medical library by the age of twelve — twice. He claimed to have taught himself eight languages. He was flying a plane at age thirteen. Much of what Jones would assert as fact might have been greeted with more skepticism — except the rest of his documented life was so outrageous.

Following a hitch in the navy during World War II — he lied about his age to enlist — he got into the business that would occupy him for decades: the exotic animal trade. Flying all over Africa, Asia, and South America, he caught snakes, crocodiles, big cats, and elephants, shipping them home in old B25 bombers to set up exhibits and compounds. He filmed hundreds of television series and documentaries — *I Search for Adventure*, *Professional Hunter*, *Capture*, ABC's *Bold Journey*, and his own series, *Wild Cargo*, which aired in February 1961.

His exploits were not confined to animals. He had shadowy ties to numerous mercenary forces, especially in Rhodesia. He likely had ties with any number of foreign and domestic intelligence agencies, including the FBI and CIA. He was even questioned about his connection to the 1963 Kennedy assassination and, in particular, David Ferrie, a CIA operative with ties to Lee Harvey Oswald and Cuban exiles, who had applied to Jones for a job as a pilot only weeks before the shooting in Dallas. The investigation of Jones went no further, though his sympathies were plain; several years prior Jones was asked if he thought Kennedy would win the presidency, and he responded, "It really doesn't matter. Some right-thinking Texan will take care of the son-of-a-bitch."

His interest in workouts and training equipment paralleled his other adventures, beginning in the late forties when a friend in Tulsa, Oklahoma, Percy Cunningham, gave him ten dollars to build a piece of equipment for the local YMCA. In 1947 he had settled for six months in California and was a regular at Vic Tanny's gym near Muscle Beach. He trained hard and went to bodybuilding shows but likely never competed, though his middle son, Gary, remembers him stating, "I made it to the stage"—suggesting he was in contests but never won. Almost from the start, Jones had toyed with the idea of a better way to lift weights. Barbells, he concluded, were inefficient because they did not correctly apply resistance through the full range of motion. He tinkered with machines for years and kept at it wherever he went, including Rhodesia, where he landed his family in the midsixties after an ill-fated film project.

It was not a great time to settle in Rhodesia, which was in the midst of political turmoil. To what extent he was involved in mercenary work is uncertain, but when the Soviet Union backed the Rhodesian opposition, he was forced to make a hasty exit. Abandoning all his assets, which the Rhodesian government confiscated, he left behind a $1.5 million cache of film, equipment, and vehicles, including a helicopter and two planes. He was $5 million in debt when he returned to the States. In Florida he rented two homes, one in DeLand, and used a $250 loan from his sister to continue working on his machines at a small welding shop. It was there that he came up with the breakthrough that would revolutionize the fitness industry.

Jones was not one to parcel out credit, though the invention owes much to his son Gary. The two had what might best be called a tense relationship. "He was a very, *very* intense person," said Gary. "He never beat us, but he was strict. We weren't allowed to speak unless we were spoken to first. If we did, we got backhanded." Gary, a math prodigy who was helping his father design the latest machine at the welding shop, had learned to stand far enough back to avoid getting hit. One night he was doing complex calculations in his head while his father worked at his design table. If Jones needed numbers, he tapped the table twice, and Gary, standing safely behind his father "so he could barely whack me," shot back the answers. They were working on a key transmission gear to vary the resistance when Gary had his sudden insight: a cam or spiral pulley. It would work more efficiently and be infinitely cheaper. When he blurted out the words *spiral pulley* without his father's permission, Jones knocked him flat. The unspoken rule was that if Gary dared to challenge his father three times, he would have earned sufficient respect to be heard. After Gary's third trip to the floor, Jones ripped off a piece of paper and told him, "Here's what I need from you. Go draw it."

Gary returned home after two in the morning and left the paper with the required dimensions on a table. The next morning Jones woke him up, but instead of driving him to school, their routine, took him to the welding shop with the blunt instruction, "Call when you're finished."

The Nautilus cam, which Gary finished designing, revolutionized the practice of exercise. Previously, a muscle was worked by the up-down lift and lowering of a weight. However, by pulling a weighted cable over a spiral-shaped cam — resembling a nautilus shell — the user experienced a varied resistance through the entire range of motion, stimulating the natural strength curve of a muscle. Variable resistance was arguably the greatest innovation in fitness equipment in the latter half of the twentieth century — but Gary's input did little to improve father-son relations.

Soon after the first Nautilus prototypes went to customers, Gary was again at the welding shop, trying to resolve an unanticipated problem. Under the stress of heavy use, the original cam had a tendency to warp. To strengthen it Gary tried forcing a thicker cam into the machine, and the machine "exploded." He woke up on top of the steel welding bench, covered in blood. When Gary got home his father greeted him at the screen door. "'What happened?' I told him the machine blew up. I had blood all over my coat. He said, 'Can you fix it?' I said, 'I don't know.' The screen door slammed, then he opened it and called me back. 'Does it hurt?' I told him no. 'It will,' he said." Gary continued, "Being raised around Arthur was different."

Not everyone was an immediate convert to Nautilus. Hard-core bodybuilders were the most suspicious, reluctant to abandon the crude iron that had worked so well in the past. For many, the Universal Machine was revolution enough. In 1974 Charles Gaines published what was then the first definitive inside look at musclemen, *Pumping Iron: The Art and Sport of Bodybuilding*. Largely anecdotal, filled with earnest profiles of the big-name competitors and key contests, it derived much of its material from a few hard-core workout meccas—primarily Gold's Gym in Venice, California. "There are also machines," wrote Gaines in describing the gym's workout floor, "even a couple of the relatively new Nautilus machines, chrome-and-Naugahyde contraptions that look like sophisticated torture devices. These are very chic machines right now. They are made by a man in Florida who claims they are revolutionizing bodybuilding. They are rarely used at Gold's. Most of the time they just sit there without the dignity of people in them, looking lonely and menacing."

Elsewhere, Nautilus was embraced with more enthusiasm. Jones evangelized at every opportunity: in exercise bulletins, in dozens of articles, at meets and events. He was a dynamic spokesperson: "Everyone was literally spellbound by the man," declared hard-core lifter Kim Wood. Even ramped-up production could barely meet demand. Bill Pearl, the bodybuilder and Oregon gym owner, lamented, "Sales of his units were going out of sight. Prospective buyers were phoning day and night to confirm what Arthur was preaching. There were so many calls, it started interfering with my ability to run my business."

Selling Nautilus, the caustic Jones had an invaluable ally in his director of research and marketing, Ellington Darden. A lifelong strength and health advocate, Darden held advanced degrees in exercise science and would go on to write more than fifty books, many promoting the Nautilus system. His partnership with Jones operated as smoothly as the Nautilus cam. "He understood what I wanted to do, and I liked him and recognized his role in the organization," said Darden. "I was one of the few who got along with him."

By the late 1970s the machines were in demand everywhere—at physical rehab centers, professional sports training centers, colleges, and high schools. The name Nautilus became the generic symbol for resistance-training machines; at gyms and clubs, prospective members invariably asked, "Do you have Nautilus?" Different machines targeted unique body parts or muscle groups, encouraging a circuit style of training. Eventually, even the biggest names in bodybuilding—Grimek, Reeves, Schwarzenegger—bought into the new technology and made the pilgrimage to meet Jones and train on Nautilus. By 1985 his company had manufactured four hundred thousand machines, generating annual sales of three hundred million dollars and landing Jones on the *Forbes* list of the four hundred richest people. Jones himself became a celebrity, appearing in magazines and on talk shows—though rarely volunteering much. Gruff, slyly combative, he stubbornly dodged an early David Letterman who peppered him with questions like, "Is it true your board meets at the International House of Pancakes?" and "What's your company worth?" and "Do you carry a gun?" "A gun is like a tourniquet," Jones replied to the last question. "Most of the time you don't need it. But when you do you want to get to it fast."

He married six times, each time to women between the ages of sixteen and twenty. His motto for summing up his favorite pursuits was "Younger women, faster airplanes, and bigger crocodiles," which was also the title of an authorized biography. He titled his autobiography *And God Laughs*. After the rented home in DeLand, he bought the six-hundred-acre Jumbolair spread, which in 1985 was home to 90 elephants, 3 rhinos, 150 snakes, and hundreds of alligators and crocodiles.

In 1986 he sold Nautilus and started the MedX Corporation to pursue research and develop even better equipment. Gary, meanwhile, had taken an increasingly important role in the company as it grew, running the main factory and briefly serving as interim president. He was not happy, however, with the new owners of Nautilus, particularly an incoming president whom he believed had a criminal record. His displeasure was not appreciated by his father, who called one day and, without introduction, told him: "'Go to Main Street and turn right. Call me from the second phone booth on the left.' I'm not making this up," said Gary. "When I called he said, 'My jet's coming to get you. Get some clothes and drive to the airport.'"

Gary flew to Jones's ranch in Ocala, where he was presented with a list of demands to join the new owner of the company. "'What am I going to get out of this?' I said, and he said, 'Nothing.' We got into a heated debate, and he said, 'What are you going to do?' I told him, 'Start my own company,' and he said, 'You don't have the balls to start your own company.' So I said, 'I guess we'll find out.'"

He had to walk into town to get a taxi to the commercial airport so he could buy a ticket home. It was the last time he and his father spoke.

Jones died twenty years later, in 2007, at the age of eighty. In one of many obituaries, Jones's younger son, William, quoted his father as saying: "I shot 630 elephants and 63 men, and I regret the elephants more." William allowed there might have been some truth to his father's claim. Anyway, he added, "You didn't argue with the man. Not twice."

Gary, meanwhile, made good on what would be his farewell words to his father. Two years after that lonely hike into town, he started a company called Hammer Strength featuring a machine he had developed that improved on the exercise motion. A practitioner of martial arts, particularly tae kwon do, Gary had long been impressed by the smooth, curved movement that went into low and high blocks. Barbells and existing machines, including Nautilus, depended on sharp, "unnatural" motion that went perpendicular to the body. Gary's innovation proved a big seller; almost overnight Hammer Strength became the number-one brand for plate-loading equipment, its manufacture aided by a highly sophisticated computer program he had developed for Hewlett-Packard. In 1997 he sold the company to Life Fitness for thirty-two million dollars.

He was not overly sentimental on the occasion of his father's death. "Arthur taught me a lot," he said. "I still read all his books and articles. But he believed in throwing you to the sharks. If you survived, he added more sharks. I didn't mind competing against the outside, but I didn't need that kind of competition from the inside. Understand, I'm not saying my dad was evil. It's just the way he was."

TWO MORE REMARKABLE MEN AND THEIR FITNESS MACHINE

Ray Wilson came from a very different background than Jones and his family of doctors. He had grown up dirt-poor during the Great Depression. The eldest of eight brothers and sisters, he had led a hardscrabble early life as part of a nomadic family that moved among the western states where Wilson's father looked for work. The family picked citrus trees in California and apricots in Colorado and baled hay on the ranches of South Dakota. The work was grueling, and life at home presented other challenges. His father was a violent man, who once knocked out his son with a chair and had brushes with the law — he burned down a bank that was foreclosing on a farm he had set up. He was also an ace mechanic, who would buy broken-down John Deere tractors that Wilson would clean with kerosene before his mother repainted them. When his father opened a used-car lot, the first of many, it was Wilson's job to find cars to sell and repossess them, occasionally, as he remembered, from a man with a gun.

To help support the family, Wilson took up life as a wrestler. He was far from the biggest man on the circuit, but he was wiry and strong and fast, a fierce competitor who never allowed himself to be pinned. It was on the wrestling circuit that he first drifted into the gyms of Salt Lake City.

Gyms in those days were still gyms, sweaty dungeons frequented mostly by bodybuilders and hard-core "muscle heads." Like Vic Tanny, he seized on the appetite for places to exercise that would appeal to a more genteel crowd. Unlike Tanny, who marketed his new upscale clubs using his name and personal glamour, Wilson stayed in the background. Never known for parceling out credit to others, he did have one partner. "The spa," Wilson admitted, "was Bob's original idea."

The "Bob" was Bob Delmonteque, a Texan who had become obsessed with weight lifting after mail-ordering a $9.95 Bob Hoffman barbell set in high school. "When the weights came," he said, "I was so excited I felt like I was having an orgasm." He signed on with the Coast Guard, worked with heavyweight champ Jack Dempsey, tried acting in Hollywood, and, with a naturopathic doctor's degree, helped a roster of Hollywood stars get fit and lose weight, among them Clark Gable, Marlon Brando, and John Wayne. In the midfifties he hooked up with Wilson, and in the next three decades they opened more than five hundred clubs.

Wilson was the impetus, an aggressive businessman with a singular talent for marketing. He was not one to back down from a challenge or miss the fun of a fight. His "American Health Studios" went toe-to-toe with Tanny in Southern California before each chain expanded nationally. "We both went kind of bananas," said Wilson. "We spent huge amounts on advertising and stole each other's people. We had a gym war. It enthused everybody, it was great for the industry, but it hurt both companies."

In Mexico, with Delmonteque riding shotgun, he developed a spa spin on another chain he had started, "Silhouette Figure Salons," and called it "European Health Spas," his strategy to attract an even more upscale clientele with luxury locker rooms, Jacuzzis, and spa amenities. At first there were alternate days for men and women, and then both sexes came together. The first club opened in California in 1960, and the chain became a huge success. Other chains would follow, and so would other "gym wars," notably one with Donahue Wildman, whose clubs would eventually anchor the Bally empire. Wilson's place in the annals of fitness is owed largely to the hundreds of clubs he started and fostered—but not entirely. He also made industry history with a machine.

The machine's origin dates to 1960 and the club Wilson opened that year, the President's Club in Houston, the city's premiere workout facility for NASA. Among its more celebrated members was astronaut James Lovell.

Lovell had a distinguished history in space. On Gemini 7, Lovell was the first astronaut to spend a fortnight out of the earth's atmosphere. After commanding Gemini 12, he had spent more time in space than any other human. In 1968 he would fly on Apollo, the first manned mission to the moon. It was Lovell, on Apollo 13, who helped save the mission—and its astronauts—after an oxygen tank exploded. He never walked on the moon, but he was only one of three men who would travel there twice.

Back on earth he was tagged to head up the President's Council on Fitness, the successor to the agency that owed its provenance to Bonnie Prudden. Lovell was a big believer in fitness, and, like Prudden, he was not happy about what he saw in the country. This was the end of the fifties, the Soviet Union was flexing its weapons muscle, and the United States needed to stay strong if it hoped to meet the global challenge. But if you looked at schools, if you checked the media, all anyone seemed to care about was smoking dope and handing out flowers.

An exception, of course, was Ray Wilson, whom he had come to know at the President's Club. Whenever Lovell went to the club he would watch Wilson work out, impressed by his physique and obsessive workout routines. Wilson was not the most charming person, but behind the tough talk and outsized ego was a decent man who kept his promises. Wilson, he knew, had made a fortune from a succession of clubs, culminating with European Health Spas, and now he was talking about the start of another operation, something called Family Fitness.

The week that Wilson invited Lovell and his son to join him on a fishing trip off Long Beach, Lovell made his pitch. He took him aside one evening. "Here's the deal," he told Wilson. "If you open more clubs and use the words *health* or *fitness* in the name or advertising, you've got to have a cardiovascular machine. If you don't, I've got the power to shut you down. And I will."

"But there is no cardiovascular machine," Wilson objected.

"Go find one," said Lovell.

In theory Wilson was all for cardiovascular training. He knew all about Dr. Paul Dudley White, who had died a few years back. A founder of the American Heart Association and renowned cardiologist, White had helped President Dwight Eisenhower recover from the heart attack he had suffered in office when everyone else despaired. The heart needed its own workout, White insisted. The pump needed exercise. You had to rev up the heartbeat. One way, maybe the most efficient way, was to work the big muscles in the legs and thighs and get the blood flowing. An excellent means to do this was biking. White was a huge believer in biking. His use of the bicycle was known throughout the world, and the seventeen-mile Dr. Paul Dudley White Bike Path in the Boston-Brookline area was named for him.

In Dallas, four hundred miles north of Houston, Dr. Kenneth Cooper was doing his own research that would lead to a whole new type of exercise that he would name "aerobics," the title of his 1968 best-selling book.

But back in 1964 there was only biking and running—on paths and tracks. Machine? What machine? thought Wilson.

He found what he was looking for on a chance visit to his sister Mary, who was living in Italy. Mary had married a race car driver, Ed Cheavers, whose dad was Mr. Arizona, an old workout buddy of Wilson and onetime driver himself who had convinced Wilson to try racing. Wilson had competed in several races, once finishing third. After a crash he decided he was allergic to the track gravel—and gave up the track for wrestling.

It was not until he was leaving Mary's house and about to jump in a cab to the airport that he thought about the strange machine he had seen in her basement. It was a big green contraption with pedals and electronic readouts, obviously designed in Italy. On impulse he ran back inside and found, to his surprise, that it was manufactured in Concord, California.

Thus began a saga that occupied — or obsessed — Wilson for the next few years. He was determined to get the "big green machine" to market. Lovell's threat made it seem as if his future depended on it.

His first setback was the factory. It was closed, though not because the machine had proved a failure. It had been designed, in fact, by Dr. Keene Dimick, the brilliant scientist who had invented gas chromography. As Wilson explained it, Dimick had spent so much time bent over peering into his microscope that he had gotten badly out of shape, so he concocted a machine to restore his health and body and called it the Lifecycle. But Dimick was a scientist, not a businessman; he gave up after losing a million dollars and sold manufacturing rights to the Oakland publisher of the military's *Stars and Stripes* newspaper. The publishing company lost another million. When Wilson showed up at its six-story building in Oakland, the company was only too happy to unload the rights — which Wilson picked up for five hundred thousand dollars.

He spent two years perfecting the machine. He sank another one hundred thousand dollars in trying to promote it. He installed the first one in his Family Fitness Center in San Diego, a club he had had started with Lance Alworth, the all-pro wide receiver for the San Diego Chargers. He assumed the machine would grab instant attention, but few seemed interested. Unfortunately, the one man who did was anything but a likely partner. He was little more than a kid, a recent graduate of nearby Claremont College, where he had opened a tiny gym. Wilson, of course, had never heard of him. Nor did his name prompt confidence. What kind of name was Augie Nieto?

Like so many men who went on to become legends in the history of fitness, Nieto had suffered miserably because of his youthful body. Unlike Charles Atlas and others tormented for their scrawny builds, Nieto was grotesquely fat. He was only five-foot-six, and in high school his weight ballooned to 265 pounds. Salesmen at clothing stores fled behind the counter when he walked in the door; at school he was sure that everyone smirked. He did not blame them. He felt like a freak. Yet he could not seem to do anything about it. When he ate he never felt full, so he kept eating. His waist was fifty-six inches. He was disgusted when he looked in the mirror. His only relief was on the football field; there, at least, size counted for something. He could not move fast, but it was hard to get around him. There was another attraction on the gridiron; she was a school cheerleader, who barely looked at him.

He went to the gym. He lifted weights. He worked out and ran. Slowly, his body changed. The pounds slid off. Fat turned to muscle. He dropped to 240, 220, 190. In the space of a year, he had lost 80 pounds. He was thrilled with the new Augie. He met the cheerleader he had had a crush on. Her name was Lynne, and she became his girlfriend. He became an apostle of exercise. "I knew that exercise was the magic pill," he said. "Once I found exercise, I wanted to spread the word."

He decided to open a gym. Nieto was then a freshman at Claremont, and he had to borrow money to start it, but he was inspired by his dad, a truck driver, who had just launched his own company. The gym was minuscule, only five hundred square feet, so small that men and women had to alternate days because there was not locker room space. He staged a fund-raiser and got forty-nine thousand dollars and replaced the weights in the gym with Nautilus equipment. What he did not have was a cardiovascular machine. "In the midseventies, the fitness industry was geared to the athlete," said Nieto. "It was biased toward strength and had nothing to do with cardiovascular exercise. I saw the opportunity to broaden the market to women at Ray Wilson's Family Fitness Center. Ray was an icon; he was a mentor to me as a young man. I learned about him from magazines. He had a great reputation for making people he worked with successful. When I saw the Lifecycle at his club I was so excited that I sold my own club and purchased the marketing rights."

He bought them for next to nothing. There was no contract, just a handshake, and Nieto loaded up his motor home with a half-dozen machines and embarked on a cross-country mission. Five thousand miles later, he had sold exactly eleven Lifecycles. He owed more than four hundred thousand dollars to family and friends. He came back to Wilson and pleaded, "Nobody wants to buy an expensive unknown machine. The only way this is going to work is if we give them away." With Wilson's reluctant approval, he identified the fifty top owners of clubs and gyms and sent them Lifecycle bikes for free. There was no commitment required. If nobody used it, fine. Nieto would pay to have it returned.

The results astonished even Nieto. Almost without exception, every club owner who took the machine bought one—or a half dozen. The factory that made the Lifecycle bike could barely keep up with orders. In the space of two years, Nieto and Wilson had sold six thousand. By the late 1970s the Lifecycle was the top-selling piece of cardio equipment in the industry.

Wilson, meanwhile, faced a dilemma: was he a club owner or equipment manufacturer? A club entrepreneur at heart, he found the Lifecycle bike something of a distraction. Plus, purchasers of the equipment were reluctant to subsidize a potential competitor in the club field, which was then beginning to boom. Together with Nieto, who stayed on in a management position, he sold the company to Bally in 1984, which renamed it Bally Life Fitness Products Corp. (later renamed Life Fitness, Inc.). The Lifecycle bike then had become a lot more complex, incorporating solid-state electronics that were computer controlled, and Bally was unique in having the required expertise to make the machine. It dominated the world of electronic console games, reaping profits from casino machines, video poker, and Pac-Man. At the same time Bally was beginning to look into club ownership. "It was," said Nieto, "the best of both worlds."

It certainly was for Nieto. Bally expanded its club interests with a spree of aggressive purchases and soon emerged as the largest club operator in the world, only to face the same dilemma as Wilson: could it juggle both running clubs and peddling equipment to rivals? In 1991 Bally resolved this conflict by selling the business to a group of senior managers that included Nieto. In 1997 Nieto sold the company again, this time to new owners Brunswick Corporation, for $310 million.

Nieto had made his name with the Lifecycle and his fortune selling it, twice. But he was much more than a deep-pocketed entrepreneur. He never forgot that exercise had changed his life, and he made it his mission to spread the word. Spared the ego of so many crusaders, as well as the caustic personality, he became a revered ambassador of fitness, traveling the world to promote a healthy lifestyle. As president of Life Fitness, he was a key early sponsor of the International Racquet and Sports Association (IRSA), then a fledgling amalgam of clubs and now the dominant trade association. He supported global events to bring the message of fitness to dozens of countries. A robust athlete, he skied and surfed and trekked around the world, often with his family—his wife, Lynne, the Claremont cheerleader, and their three children.

Ultimately, neither wealth nor his status in the fitness community would spare him from a fate that made his devotion to exercise seem a terrible irony.

As for the Lifecycle, it ultimately became enshrined near O'Hare Airport in Chicago, the headquarters of Life Fitness. The very first model is on display there in a glass case. Atop a sturdy if ungainly pedaling frame, a multidial box is bracketed to the handlebars—"the exclusive computer coach," reads the promo brochure. A shapely woman in a black leotard stands with a finger aimed at one of the dials while the copy promises: "Puts you in tip top Physical Condition . . . and keeps you there!"

Anchored by the Lifecycle, Life Fitness emerged as the global leader in fitness equipment, with multiple lines of treadmills, bikes, and strength equipment. In a serendipitous twist, the company also bought Hammer Strength, the business of Gary Jones, thus bringing under one roof the two pioneers of the machine age—Arthur Jones and Ray Wilson.

THE REBEL AND HIS REFORMER

There was, it needs noting, another machine that had gained a measure of notoriety in the 1960s. A long, narrow slab of wood with straps and pulleys, it resembled less a machine than a medieval torture device, and its ominous-sounding name, "The Reformer," did not help. The contraption was not to be found in any of the day's clubs and gyms. For the true believers, there was only one place to partake of its benefits: a spacious if dimly lit second-floor loft on Lower Eighth Avenue in New York City. There, clients spent hours flat on their backs or exercising on mats while the man who invented the machine barked gruff commands. Even those unfamiliar with his name or work would have stopped to stare if they happened to be passing along the sidewalk outside on a wintry day and spotted the octogenarian taking a brisk walk between sessions, dressed in his training bikini and smoking a fat cigar. The man was Joseph Pilates.

Today, a half century later, Pilates is a global exercise brand. Most major health clubs offer Pilates classes. Few cities of any size lack Pilates studios or trainers schooled in the Pilates Method. Most "fusion" classes incorporate Pilates. Worldwide, upwards of fifteen million people devote hours each week on "The Reformer" or repeating the exercises their inventor devised. Pilates himself famously said, "My work is fifty years ahead of its time," and history has proved him right.

He was born in a small village near Düsseldorf, Germany, in 1880, the son of a prizewinning gymnast and a mother who was a naturopath. A sickly child, he suffered from asthma, rickets, and rheumatic fever and often endured the taunts of bullies. In one harrowing episode he was pounded on the head with a rock, leaving him virtually blind in the left eye for the rest of his life. Determined to restore his health and confidence, he studied yoga and martial arts. He became engrossed in anatomy, poring over books and, legend has it, hiding in the woods near his home to watch how animals moved their muscles. He boxed and taught self-defense and performed as a gymnast. In 1912 he moved to England, either (there are two stories) to box or to tour with a circus, posing with his brother in a Greek-statue act. He taught self-defense at public schools and at Scotland Yard.

When war broke out in 1914 he was interned along with other German nationals in a camp for enemy aliens in Lancaster, England, and used the opportunity to promote his fitness program. Transferred to a second camp on the Isle of Man, he worked in the infirmary for the most grievously injured soldiers, devising a method of exercise by rigging mattress springs and attaching them to bedposts. No photos exist of the makeshift devices, but they were likely the basis for his system of exercises that he would later call "Contrology."

Or so fable has it. A great deal of myth surrounds Pilates's early life, much of it a mix of cherished anecdote and repeated error. Dedicated researchers, most of them longtime Pilates teachers, have sparred for years to separate fact from fiction. Oft-cited evidence of his miraculous holistic approach to exercise was the great 1918 influenza epidemic. Though it ravaged tight-knit communities of people, such as those in internment camps, supposedly none who practiced Pilates's method in England fell fatally ill.

The reason for his emigration to the United States is likewise a topic of debate. One version lays the motive to his disaffection with the government: back in Germany after the war, he had taught self-defense to the Hamburg Military Police and was then asked to train the army in 1925 but balked because he did not approve of the political direction

Germany was taking. Another version, likely factual, stresses his planned new life across the Atlantic: he shipped off to train boxers at the behest of a friend, Nat Fleischer, the new president of *Ring* magazine, himself a pal of heavyweight Max Schmelling (whom Pilates was later rumored to train).

Whatever prompted him to leave Germany, the crossing to New York in 1926 was a momentous event in Pilates's life. It was on the ship *Westphalia* that he met his wife Clara. Or so goes the story. One of the more dogged Pilates researchers has pored over records and found no indication the two were ever married. Pilates then was already married — to his second wife, Elfriede. Applying for U.S. citizenship in 1939, Pilates declared that he and Elfriede remained married until her death in 1931. In the same document he also declared himself a widower, naming a first wife, Maria, who died in 1913 and was the mother of his daughter, Leni. Nor is it absolutely certain what Clara did. Their shipboard romance has it that Pilates fell in love with Clara, a nurse, but the word *nurse* — as listed in the Ellis Island records — was likely mistranslated. Clara actually wrote that she worked in a "nursery" — meaning she was a nanny. There is even indication — courtesy of another researcher, who found ship manifests — that Pilates had made a previous trip the year before, traveling first class, to meet with the patent attorneys who would later trademark his inventions.

Undisputed is the fact that Pilates took up residence at 939 Eighth Avenue, likely because of its proximity to the old Madison Square Garden, where boxing was becoming popular. Or — perhaps by design — he picked the building, a former gym, because it housed dance studios and rehearsal spaces. This was the early thirties, the star-studded years when modern dance and ballet were about to enjoy a heyday in America, and Pilates was quick to use the space to promote his specialty, rehabilitation. Soon the most famous names in dance — Martha Graham, Ted Shawn, George Balanchine, Jerome Robbins — were packing their injured dancers off to "Uncle Joe" to get fixed.

His skill at working with injuries earned him a fast-growing clientele, including members of the Gimbel and Guggenheim families and movie stars such as Vivien Leigh, Laurence Olivier, and Katharine Hepburn. But Pilates was much more than a rehab man. The appeal of his method, then and since, was its fusion of rigorous exercises with the promise of ultimate control — of the body and spirit. Health, he believed, was the natural human state, corrupted only by the ills of civilization. The best way to restore vitality was through "Contrology." "Contrology is a complete coordination of body, mind and spirit," he wrote in his book *Return to Life through Contrology*. "Through Contrology you first purposefully acquire complete control of your own body and then through proper repetition of its exercises you gradually and progressively acquire that natural rhythm and coordination associated with all your subconscious activities."

Faithfully perform the exercises, Pilates promised, and you will attain grace, endurance, power, even mastery of the mind. Dormant areas of the brain will spring to life. The heart will be rejuvenated, senses aroused, willpower restored. Ever grandiloquent, a born primitive, he spared no metaphor in extolling the miracle of his work: "As the spring freshets born of the heavy rains and vast masses of melting snows on mountains in the hinterlands cause rivers to swell and rush turbulently onward to the sea, so too will your blood flow with renewed vigor as the direct result of your faithfully performing the Contrology exercises."

The floridity of his language was complemented by the rigor of his work. He taught no classes; he instructed only one-on-one. His manner was brisk and authoritarian. Clients were required to be committed to his exercises and to work hard; if they did not, they were shown the door. His eccentric costume — white swimming trunks and canvas sneakers — belied the no-nonsense atmosphere of the studio. He concluded sessions with the barked, "One hour! Hit zee shower!" If the client needed guidance in skin care — of utmost importance, believed Pilates — he was not averse to joining them in the shower to demonstrate how to use the hard-bristled scrubbing brush.

Few ascribed any ulterior motive to these shower visits, though Pilates did have his fun-loving side. He enjoyed whiskey and Cuban cigars. The work ethic in the studio notwithstanding, he was a lively fixture at parties, and the good times may have extended to the living space at 939 Eighth Avenue. Mary Bowen, one of his early students, was quite certain that Pilates, Clara, and another resident in the loft enjoyed an intimate ménage à trois.

He wrote two books: *Your Health* in 1934 and *Return to Life through Contrology* in 1945. In the latter he reiterated his belief that the world would be a far better place, free of suffering, if his methods were adopted. He promoted his work wherever he could: he created exercise pamphlets, taught at armed forces bases, even sold his equipment on Saturdays at Macy's. Aside from "The Reformer" and assorted strap devices, this included the Wunda Chair, a comfy armchair that could be tilted ninety degrees and resistance springs attached to the seat. Exercisers could then use the levered seat to perform a full-body workout, ranging from bends and presses to what looks uncannily like the Stair Master, a machine that would not be invented for forty years.

Every summer he and Clara went to Jacob's Pillow, a renowned dance retreat in the Berkshire Mountains. There he led group exercise classes on the spacious lawns or supervised freewheeling duets on the "Dancers' Dock" that overlooked an Edenic lake. As seen in vintage 8mm film, the summer idylls offered a more relaxed atmosphere with lively sessions of "head wrestling" – a kind of Sumo exercise with Pilates and friends such as Shawn, hands behind backs, pushing each other's padded foreheads to knock the opponent off his feet.

His core clientele were dancers, but he worked with anybody who had suffered an injury or whose body needed repair. Many polio victims showed up at the loft on Eighth Avenue, as did athletes and socialites, and he invented machines to help them. Physical therapy as a discipline did not exist then, and Pilates was eager to demonstrate the unique value of his exercises. Hearing of President Kennedy's back problems, he repeatedly sought a visit to the White House – to no avail.

Neither presidents nor the general citizenry were ready to embrace his philosophy or apparatus. He won some credence when the chief of orthopedics at Lenox Hill Hospital endorsed his methods, which were gaining modest traction when, in 1966, a fire broke out in the loft on Eighth Avenue. Attempting to salvage what he could, Pilates fell through the burned-out floorboards and had to hang by his hands from a beam until rescued by firefighters. The trauma contributed to his death the following year at age eighty-seven, or so – again – legend has it. Bowen, for one, dismissed this account as "ridiculous." "There was a fire in the storeroom," she said. "The next day Joe came in to check the damage, and his leg went through a hole in the floor. [That] was his only injury. Business went right on. He only started to get ill two years later, complaining to Clara, 'I can't breathe.'" According to Bowen, his failing health was due to emphysema and cigars, which he took up to compensate for the overwhelming disappointment in his life—that he was not taken more seriously. "Two days before he died, [a friend] went to visit him, and he was angry, very angry, angry about his body, angry about his life. Fitness arrived in the U.S. in the seventies," said Bowen, "too late for Joe, who died in 1967—disillusioned with all of us."

Had he lived another five or ten years, he might have taken some comfort from the beginnings of more widespread acceptance, in particular the embrace of Hollywood stars. In the spring of 1972 one of his original acolytes, Ron Fletcher, opened a West Coast studio on Rodeo Drive at Wilshire Boulevard. Fletcher had danced with Martha Graham and went on to Broadway as a choreographer before moving west, and his Beverly Hills studio quickly became the favored workout space for a cluster of actresses, among them Ali MacGraw, Barbra Streisand, Candice Bergen, and Katharine Ross. Studio executives came by, as did celebrities and members of Hollywood high society; Nancy Reagan was a regular.

Fletcher held particular authority because he was one of only a few Pilates teachers who could claim direct ties to the great man himself, a small group known reverentially as "the Elders." But despite the burst of star power from Fletcher, despite its quietly growing recognition, it would be another quarter century before Pilates became the phenomenon it is today. That development would happen only as the result of a bitter legal battle and an epic trademark suit at the start of the new millennium.

CHAPTER 5

Gotta Move, 1960s–1980s

Ken Cooper rouses the country with "aerobics"; Jim Fixx sells the "runner's high"; women take control; the Sultan of Sweat; the shoe wars get into step

DOING THE COOPER

Bowen was right in characterizing the 1970s as the decade when "fitness started in the U.S.," though one might better date its genesis to the late 1960s when a new habit of exercise became the rage in America. By most any account, the sixties were an unlikely time for the start of a fitness craze. The media were entranced with the youth culture and the hippie movement. The prevailing mantra was "sex, drugs, and rock and roll." Young men who were not off fighting in Vietnam were parading with "Peace and Love" placards. Long hair was in; exercise was definitely out. Those who paid attention to what they ate and what they did with their bodies were scorned as "health nuts." Few adults bothered much with muscles. Men wanted to look like George Harrison and act like Keith Richards; for women, the prevailing fashion model was Twiggy. "The sophisticated life, as portrayed in books and movies, described so vividly by writers like John Cheever," declared *New York Times* science reporter Gina Kolata, "featured cigarettes and cocktails before dinner, not a sweaty session in a gym or on a tennis court or a five-mile run."

If there was any keen interest in the body, it was its weightlessness in space, which is what Dr. Kenneth Cooper was studying in the 1960s. An air force flight surgeon, he was director of the Aerospace Medical Laboratory in San Antonio, conditioning astronauts to help them overcome the debilitating effects of a zero-gravity atmosphere.

Cooper loved to fly and had dreamed of becoming an astronaut himself. He was also preoccupied with exercise, an interest sparked by his own health scare. He had been a star all-state athlete in track and basketball at the University of Oklahoma, which did not please his father, who worried his son would succumb to "athlete's heart"—a feared cause of early death in the 1950s. His mother rarely missed a game or meet, but Cooper's involvement with sports came to a halt during medical school when he watched his weight balloon. Inactive for years, he went water skiing at age twenty-nine and suffered an acute episode of tachycardia. "I thought I was having a heart attack. I got nauseous, lightheaded; my heart rate shot up. At the hospital the doctor told me, 'The only thing wrong with you is you're out of shape.' It's what shoved me back to reality."

He started exercising again. He began eating healthy. He dropped the forty pounds he had gained in medical school and, within a year, ran his first marathon. He was the last finisher and would not have officially finished at all had his wife, Millie, not convinced race officials to wait around to clock his time. (It was 6:24.) This inauspicious debut did not deter Cooper, who today likes to boast, "Forty-four years later, I've run thirty-eight thousand miles." Nor did it alter his new career plan. He was now committed to preventive medicine, even though "in medical school we were taught to avoid the specialty of preventive medicine because there was no profit in health; the profit was in disease."

He returned to San Antonio and a residency in the aerospace medicine program where the chance remark of a classmate forever changed his life. "We should be able to measure the benefits of exercise like we can measure the benefits of antibiotics," said his friend. "Why don't we know the dose of exercise to prescribe to people?"

It was, said Cooper, "like a switch flipped in my head."

In San Antonio he began a rigorous study of what being "in shape" meant. Tasked with getting astronauts in top condition, he rated activities—swimming, cycling, running, walking—based on how much oxygen the heart pumped to the body. He conducted field tests and bed-rest studies to simulate weightlessness. He ran tests on treadmills. All the information culminated in the creation of a twelve-minute test to gauge aerobic capacity; running less than a mile rated "very poor"; running 1.75 miles qualified as "excellent." He assigned points to each exercise routine and came up with goals needed to get and stay fit. He declared a benchmark of thirty points a week after a sixteen-week program.

When a journalist, Kevin Brown, interviewed him for the Sunday supplement of *Family Weekly*, a feature called, "How to Exercise the Astronaut Way," he and Brown decided to collaborate on a book. It took two years of writing and editing. Near the end of the process, Cooper, Brown, and the publisher were discussing the first chapter in the publisher's New York office. He had labeled it "aerobic," using the adjective that meant literally "living on air," then added an *s* to invent a noun to describe the exercise program. "My publisher said, 'Let's call the entire book *Aerobics*.' I told him that's not a good idea. People can't pronounce it. They won't be able to spell it. No one will remember it."

Cooper's book *Aerobics* came out in 1968 and stayed on the *New York Times* best-seller list for eleven weeks. It went on to sell thirty million copies and has been translated into forty-one languages. It was not, however, greeted with instant acclaim. Cooper liked to tell the tale of an early promotion fiasco with Barbara Walters, who was interviewing him for her radio program, *Monitor*. Walters strolled into the green room, her hair in curlers, and ignored him. "What is wrong with you?" he demanded, and she retorted, "You're a fraud. I called air force headquarters and they said they don't support your book or programs." Cooper whipped out his research on twenty-seven thousand servicemen and insisted Walters call again. She did and returned to book him on *The Today Show*, where she was cohost.

It was the start of a media blitz that made Cooper famous but also made him think twice about his career in the military. The first dream to go was flying into space as an astronaut. "I saw how I was making a difference here at home," he decided, "and helping people meant keeping my feet on earth." Then came another defining crossroads: he was offered a fast track to becoming a commander of an air force hospital. He was forty years old then, a lieutenant colonel, and needed the posting to reach the rank of full colonel. "It was total idiocy. I told them, 'Let me stay in San Antonio and continue my work.' I had a whole research lab. I could care less about a promotion. I had thirteen years in the military. In several years I could retire; there was the possibility of becoming surgeon general, so they said. I had to make a decision, and I did. I walked away then with a pregnant wife, a five-year-old daughter, and the prospect of no insurance, and moved to Dallas. It was a huge gamble."

In Dallas in 1970, he opened a small two-room office and saw his first patient as a preventive-medicine physician. Months later he was called before the Dallas County Medical Society, which was alarmed that his treadmill stress test would give people heart attacks. "The board thought I was going to kill people," said Cooper. "They were trying to run me out of town." Once again he pulled out his data, so convincing the board chairman that the man became the second physician to perform the stress test on patients in Dallas.

His stubborn tenacity served him well and did much the same for aerobics and the study of healthy living. In Dallas he founded the Cooper Aerobics Center, a thirty-acre campus that would come to employ six hundred people and run on a budget of sixty-five million dollars. He would write more than a dozen books. His collaboration with PepsiCo spurred an international effort to eliminate trans fats; on the back of Baked Lay packages he was quoted: "Fitness is a journey, not a destination. It must be continued for the rest of your life." His twelve-minute standard became widespread in the world of athletics. It remains the test for international soccer referees and linesmen, who must run a certain distance to qualify; in Brazil, where he trained the 1970 soccer team to a World Cup win, running is still called "coopering" or "doing the cooper."

Dogged if not dogmatic, he never abandoned or even modified his earliest pronouncements, but he did, in time, shift a few priorities. In *Aerobics* he was skeptical of the female interest in fitness and cited a Seattle woman who told him after a lecture, "Doctor, I don't care about the heart and the lungs and all that. I just want some sweet little exercise that will keep my tummy tucked in." He let that remark go without comment but was duly disdainful in 1972 when his wife published her own book and was asked on a television talk show: "Is it ladylike to swim?" In 2011 he proudly declared, "Last year there were half a million marathon participants, and 52 percent were women. Women now lead the country."

Increasingly, he evangelized for older people exercising and devised numbers to adjust the balance between a focus on muscle conditioning and aerobics. As Cooper himself aged, he urged the elderly to prioritize modest strength training to counter the loss of muscle mass (reversing the ratio he prescribed for a person in their twenties, who needed an 80 percent focus on aerobics). He had strict guidelines for anyone who wanted to slow down the aging process, which mandated no cigarettes, limited alcohol, proper nutrition, and a generous dose of exercise. "If you can, walk at 3.5 miles an hour—that's a seventeen-minute mile. Walking speed is the best predictor of longevity."

JIM FIXX SELLS THE "RUNNER'S HIGH"

For all its notoriety, the publication of *Aerobics* in 1968 was not the only event that year to herald a new awareness about running—or track. The Olympics were held that summer in Mexico City. The Black Power salutes by two African American sprinters—Tommie Smith and John Carlos—during the 200-meter medal ceremony stole much of the headlines, but there were other American records in the thin air. Al Oerter won a fourth consecutive gold in the discus; Bob Beamon leaped an astonishing 29.2 feet in the long jump; Dick Fosbury took gold in the high jump with his famous, and soon to be standard, "Fosbury Flop."

At the University of Oregon, meanwhile, the most exciting long-distance runner of his day, Steve Prefontaine, was igniting a new passion for the sport. Matinee-idol handsome, with equal parts arrogance and talent, he buried the competition whenever he took to the track or cross-country route. With his blistering front-running strategy, he set American records in every distance from 2 miles through 10,000 meters. His coach was Bill Bowerman, with whom he had a testy relationship and who would go on to design the famous Nike "waffle-sole" shoe, and together the two set their sights on the 1972 Olympics in Munich, their goal to unseat the great Finnish champion, Lassi Virrin, in the 10K.

The Munich Olympics were marred by the tragic slaughter of Israeli athletes by a band of Arab terrorists, and Prefontaine, in a furious duel, was outkicked by Virrin and ended finishing a disappointing fourth. But the 1972 Olympics were noteworthy for a singular American triumph: Frank Shorter won the marathon.

Shorter had been Prefontaine's longtime training partner—in fact, he was the second-to-last person to see him alive the night Prefontaine died in a car crash only months after Munich. He had won the U.S. national cross-country championships four years in a row (1970–73), but it was his marathon win that secured his place in history. He took a silver medal in the 1976 Olympics marathon in Montreal—and remains the only American to medal twice in the Games' marquee event. Soon after he abruptly retired from competitive running and went on to pursue a career in law. He became a frequent commentator on televised sports and headed up the United States Anti-Doping Agency. He made headlines again in 2011 when he revealed a traumatic childhood, the result of an abusive belt-wielding father.

Shorter galvanized interest in long-distance running, but he was not alone. In the quiet little town of Rumson, New Jersey, neighbors of George Sheehan were bewildered to spot the middle-aged cardiologist do obsessive laps around a dirt track in his backyard. They were further astonished when the doctor took to the streets during lunch breaks, pounding the river road in long johns and a ski mask. Sheehan's own family was not sure what made George run. "'Why does your father run around town in his underwear' we children were asked," said Sheehan's son Andrew. "I recall being unable to answer—recall, too, a touch of embarrassment."

Sheehan himself was anything but embarrassed. The Catholic father of twelve children, he had a busy medical practice, friends, tennis pals, a devoted wife—but his patients were driving him crazy, a condition he would later attribute to "middle-age melancholia."

"Being a doctor's not a big deal," he once explained, addressing the psychiatric staff at New York's Montefiore Hospital. "What do you hear? Constipation followed by backache followed by depression followed by hypertension followed by constipation and backache. Eight hours of that and you've *got* to get out on the road!"

At age forty-five, he revived a college passion as a star miler. In appearance he was an ungainly runner, flapping his arms like a bird, and the effort took its toll. "When he first started," said his wife, Mary Jane, "it was agony. He was in bed for three hours, completely doubled over with cramps."

But he persevered. At age forty-eight he ran the first of twenty-one consecutive Boston Marathons. At age fifty he set a world age-group record for the mile of 4:47. He began writing books, most notably *Dr. Sheehan on Running* and *Running and Being: The Total Experience*. He was the medical editor of *Runner's World* magazine and wrote dozens of columns. He spoke constantly—to corporations, conventions, and runners' groups. Up on the podium he was the sport's philosopher-king, part ham, part monk; his talks were nonstop entertainments, a stream of Kant, Descartes, and Casey Stengel, all peppered with Sheehan's erudite wit and delight in the power of shock. A log of one hour-long talk (as always, without notes) showed him quoting forty philosophers, historians, and writers, ranging from Cervantes and Tolstoy to Jung. "When I run the roads, I am a saint," he wrote. "For that hour, I am an Assisi wearing the least and meanest of clothes. I am Gandhi, the young London law student, trotting 10 to 12 miles a day and then going to a cheap restaurant to eat his fill of bread. I am Thoreau, the solitary seeking union with the world around him."

Going the Distance, his last book, was published shortly after his death from prostate cancer in 1993. Sheehan's books and a *Runner's World* column—"When the Stress of Modern Living Becomes Too Much, Run"—are listed in the hefty bibliography of another more famous writer who landed running, and himself, on the cover of every celebrity magazine and morning-television talk show. It was not false modesty when the author quoted the editor of the *Runner*, who told him: "Frank Shorter invented running. You invented the running book." The book was *The Complete Book of Running* by Jim Fixx. It featured a bright-red cover with nothing on it but the author's tanned, lean-muscled legs.

Fixx published his book in 1977, and it quickly shot to the top of the *Times* best-seller list. Bookstores could not keep it in stock. The media clamored for interviews. American Express flew Fixx to Paris on the Concorde to film commercials. Companies begged for his endorsement. Famous actors buttonholed him for interviews. So did authors and politicians. President Jimmy Carter collapsed during a 10,000-meter race near Camp David and was baffled by the mishap; he had trained, he explained, according to principles in *The Complete Book of Running*.

Fixx's celebrity catapulted jogging into a national pastime. The magazine *Runner's World*, founded in 1966, saw its circulation rocket from thirty-five thousand in 1975 to more than two hundred thousand in 1978. The National Jogging Association reported that membership jumped to twenty thousand in 1978—up from eight thousand the year before. Fixx's reign as the rock star of running lasted long past his next best seller—*Jim Fixx's Second Book of Running*—and so surprised Fixx that he went on to write a third book, *Jackpot!*, to chronicle his life in what the cover blurb called "The Great American Fame Machine."

Prior to bursting into the spotlight, there had not been much remarkable in Fixx's life. A respected magazine editor (at *McCall's*, *Life*, and *Horizon*), he was a member of the Mensa high-IQ club and had authored three books on puzzles. He was also in terrible shape—a two-pack-a-day smoker who weighed 240 pounds. He started running to repair a calf muscle he had pulled on a tennis court. They were casual runs, a mile here or there, but within weeks he noticed a change. He lost weight (he would eventually drop sixty pounds), he cut back on drinking, and he felt energized. "I noticed some surprising psychological benefits as well. I was calmer, less readily stressed by crisis and pressure. I felt cheerful, buoyant and optimistic. Work seemed easier and play more fun. In short, I suspected that there was more to running than most people, even most experts, knew."

What started out as a quick book—"breezy and superficial"—to supplement his income turned into a massive research project. He read everything that had been written on running and interviewed dozens of experts (though not Frank Shorter, who never returned his phone calls). By the time it was published, he was not only a committed runner, with fast times in two Boston Marathons, but the world's authority on the sport. His breezy, no-nonsense style coupled with detailed advice on shoes, clothes, races, injuries, and physiology prompted dozens of reviewers to tag it "the jogger's bible."

He was less a prophet when it came to nutrition. His weight had ballooned on burgers and milkshakes, and there were reports he continued to eat fast food. The alarms about fat, given widespread publicity by low-fat maven Nathan Pritikin, made little impression on Fixx, and he insisted that any nonsmoker who could run a marathon in under four hours enjoyed immunity from having a heart attack, no matter his diet. He even telephoned Pritikin to protest his chapter in *The Pritikin Promise* titled "Run and Die on the American Diet," calling it "hysterical."

Fixx himself seemed in tip-top shape, even if he did sneak donuts and burgers, an exemplar of the running lifestyle. As distinct from Cooper, whose attitude tended toward stern reproach, Fixx was a passionate but amiable preacher. He brought a common man's zeal to the road and track, convincing millions of Americans that running was the ideal pursuit to achieve health and fitness, a virtual guarantee of a longer, happier life. It thus produced a nationwide shock when a motorcyclist in northern Vermont stopped his bike at the side of a road when he noticed a body—and found Jim Fixx.

Fixx became almost as famous in death as he had in life. An autopsy confirmed he had died of a heart attack and revealed that three of his arteries were almost completely blocked by plaque, a chronic condition known as "atherosclerosis." He was fifty-two years old and badly in need of a bypass. Apologists insisted that running, far from killing him, had likely prolonged his life. The man had died in the midst of his daily jog—doing what he loved. Those who had remained skeptical of the miraculous benefits of running (there were a few) found his death a lesson in hubris. He had paid the price for his claims to invincibility, for his celebrity, for his refusal to alter his diet. Cooper, the man of science, took a detailed look at his medical records, interviewed friends and family, and ended by publishing a list of risk factors that likely contributed to his death: longtime smoker, stress (that high-flying lifestyle, two divorces), enlarged heart, and genetics (Fixx's father had died of a heart attack at age forty-three). Eventually, the furor died down, leaving everyone with a sober truism. Exercise was great, running especially so, but you still had to watch what you ate . . . and maybe see a doctor.

WOMEN GET INTO THE ACT

The bold-face names that launched the jogging boom were all men. Though Cooper would later coauthor a book with his wife, *Aerobics for Women*, his nod to females in *Aerobics* was at best minimal and at worst sexist. "It's your health, and health has no sex," he wrote, and went on to recommend running as the "best and quickest way to work up a worthwhile sweat and get your points. . . . If running is not your cup of tea, however, swimming is second best and definitely ladylike. You can wear your pretty bathing suit and socialize around the pool."

Such remarks were not greeted with enthusiasm by the rising tide of feminists, who were beginning to have a profound impact at the time *Aerobics* was published. In 1963 Betty Friedan had published her landmark book, *The Feminine Mystique*, which questioned the dominant ideology that women's fulfillment lay primarily in marriage and motherhood. In 1966 the National Organization for Women was founded, and Friedan was elected its first president. In 1972 Gloria Steinem cofounded *Ms. Magazine*, the first mass-market periodical aimed at women who demanded equality and power. That same year Title VII of the Civil Rights Act was amended to cover educational institutions, previously excluded; known as Title IX, it had a giant impact on school athletics, which were now compelled to give women equal opportunity.

It was against this background that women came to play a major, if not dominant, role in exercise, notably in the area of aerobics. The women who invented the two most famous programs were, like almost everyone, dancers. They were virtual contemporaries, though, remarkably, each operated totally independently. There is no evidence they ever met.

Foremost among them was Jacki Sorenson, the founder of Aerobic Dance. Born Jackie Faye Mills in Oakland, California, in 1942, she got the dancing bug early: at age twelve she taught her first class; at sixteen she was dancing professionally. She opted for college instead of a career onstage, and then followed the lead of her husband, Neil Sorenson, who was in the air force. When Neil was assigned to a base in Texas, she became a partner in a local dance school and a Dallas Cowboys cheerleader; when he got transferred to a base in Sacramento and then Puerto Rico, she taught dance to the airmen's wives. A fan of *Aerobics*, she wrote to Cooper, who suggested she give the wives his twelve-minute test. In 1969 she started a live show on the base's television station and called it *Aerobic Dancing*.

Its growth into a hugely successful business took years, much of it tracking the geography of her husband's job shifts (he left the air force in 1970 and went into aviation insurance). Wherever she found herself she taught classes — to teenagers, at colleges, at YMCAs. She ran workshops for students, who taught at schools and churches and more YMCAs. She updated her choreography and music for designated students (she called them "clinicians"), who held "clinics" for Aerobic Dance instructors who, in turn, started classes in other cities. Some marched in holiday parades or did halftime shows at sports events or joined Sorenson in hosting danceathons. There was no marketing, no television, virtually no advertising; instead, it was a great groundswell of interest spread only by word of mouth and demonstrations, which reached epic proportions with costumed shows at hotels and resorts.

The media jumped onboard in 1979 when Sorenson published her first book, *Aerobic Dancing*, and did a cross-country tour to promote it, appearing on dozens of news and television talk shows. The following year she released a record album to accompany the book, as well as audio and videocassette tapes. In 1981 her company, Aerobic Dancing, Inc. (ADI), had grown to more than four thousand certified instructors, seventy superinstructors (the "clinicians"), and platoons of employees who ran fifteen hundred field offices in forty-five states.

That would be its peak. Before the decade ended, ADI would declare bankruptcy and reemerge as Jacki's, Inc., with a skeleton staff of seven. The collapse of the business was due to several factors. Class size was limited, because Sorenson wanted plenty of room for her elaborate routines. ADI instructors left the nonprofit YMCAs, the source of so much early excitement, to gain more control and better compensation. ADI paid only hourly wages and never started a franchise system that retained loyalty and encouraged entrepreneurship — unlike Jazzercise, a program that came to dominate the competition and turned its more commercially savvy founder, Judi Sheppard Missett, into a group-fitness icon.

Born Judi Sheppard two years after Sorenson, in 1944, Missett (she would marry Jack Missett, a television news reporter) grew up in small-town Iowa, another dance prodigy. Her mother hired instructors to commute to their home, where she recruited other students and set up studio space. Missett was teaching dance at ten and touring professionally at age fourteen. A speech major at Northwestern University, she began teaching jazz dance in Chicago after graduating but quickly realized her students were not there to start a career — they wanted to lose weight and have a good time. She got the idea to incorporate exercise, put on snappy upbeat music, and had her class turn their backs on the mirror and dance "just for fun." In 1974 she changed the name "Dance Just for Fun" to "Jazzercise," a name suggested by one of her students in Carlsbad, California, where she had moved.

What set her apart from Sorenson was her decision to audition and train instructors, then send them out as independent contractors who would pay Jazzercise a percentage of fees or profits. At a time when Aerobic Dance instructors were being paid eight to ten dollars an hour, Jazzercise instructors were making thirty-five and forty dollars. Several celebrity fans, among them the wife of the Cleveland Browns' star quarterback, Brian Sipe, gave her a big publicity boost. To spread the word, she made revolutionary use of a video camera to replace written notes of her fast-changing routines and bought VCR machines, relatively new then, to sell to her far-flung instructors. Her book *Jazzercise: A Fun Way to Fitness* was published in 1978 — the same year as Fixx's first book — and sold more than four hundred thousand copies.

She made business news, too. Missett was instrumental in changing California's franchise laws in 1983 to enable her Jazzercise instructors to officially become franchisees, and Jazzercise was regularly listed as one of the top twenty-five U.S. franchises by the magazine *Franchise*. Jazzercise instructors performed at the opening ceremonies of the 1984 Olympics in Los Angeles. In 1986 President Ronald Reagan hailed her as one of the country's top women entrepreneurs.

Sorenson and Missett were the two high-profile innovators, the reigning queens of aerobic fitness, but there were others, a few who predated them. A woman named Martha Rounds was big on Slimnastics — a likely variant of LaLanne's "Trimnastics" — and mixed stretches and calisthenics with big-band music, adding dance routines when aerobics became popular. Her students were mostly women who came to lose weight and firm up their bodies. Two sisters, Debbie Rosas and Jennifer Rosas, formed the Bod Squad, big in the Bay Area, and later pioneered low-impact aerobics with floor routines grounded in yoga and the martial arts. Arden Zin was a follower of Bonnie Prudden, traveling with Prudden to demonstrate her exercises while Prudden lectured, and founded "Ardenics." Nancy Strong, another Prudden acolyte — she was her neighbor in White Plains — launched Aerobic Slimnastics. A contemporary, Sheila Cluff, counted both Prudden and Cooper as mentors and came up with "Cardio-Vascular Dancing" (referred to as CV Dancing) and opened up health resorts in the Los Angeles area.

California, the nation's trend capital for fitness, was also the launch pad for Gilda Marx. (Born Gilda Wilstein, she married Robert Marx, the son of the Marx Brothers' Gummo.) Yet another dancer, she started classes in a small studio in the back of a beauty salon in Encino — a mix of jazz dance, stretches, yoga, and muscle work, with popular music on the stereo — and soon everyone was talking about "Gilda from Encino." Shirley MacLaine hired her as a personal trainer. Marx moved operations to Beverly Hills, changed the name to "Body Design by Gilda," and then opened three studios in New York City. Barbra Streisand was such a fan that she included a sequence of a Marx teaching class in her 1979 film, *The Main Event*. Unhappy with the prevailing exercise gear, Marx designed a best-selling line of bright, flexible leotards made of Lycra and started a company, Flexatard, which revolutionized the dancewear industry. The high point, or low point, of her career was the day a young woman stopped by her Century City studio, started scribbling notes, and then inquired where she got her exercise mats and barres. Marx asked why she wanted to know, and the woman answered: "I'm working for Jane Fonda."

FEELING THE BURN

In many ways Fonda was the unlikeliest of models for women. She had struggled throughout her early life to escape the shadow of her father, Henry Fonda. The iconic star of films such as *Grapes of Wrath*, *Abe Lincoln*, and *Twelve Angry Men*, Fonda projected a folksy but granite image of masculinity, determined to stand up for what was right and true. At home he was very different. As described by his daughter in her autobiography, *My Life So Far*, her father was a tightly coiled, bitter man who flew into frightening rages and was incapable of warmth or support. To compensate for the lack of affirmation, she became a bulimic, bingeing and purging to achieve what she imagined would be the perfect body. It would remain a secret addiction, hidden from friends and family, well into her forties.

An undergraduate at Vassar, she fled the collegiate life and departed, on a whim, for Paris, where she modeled and studied art. It was there that she met bad-boy French filmmaker Roger Vadim, who had burst onto the scene with *And God Created Woman*, featuring his sexpot lover, Brigitte Bardot.

Returning to the States, she joined the Actors Studio, the intense gut workshop where Lee Strasberg presided over the likes of Marlon Brando, Marilyn Monroe, and Al Pacino. It was the perfect place for Fonda to hone her talent and exorcise family demons — her cold, remote dad; her mom who slashed her throat in a psychiatric hospital (for years Fonda was told she had died of a heart attack). She appeared on Broadway to mixed reviews and made her debut film, *Tall Story*, in 1960. Her breakthrough role came in *Cat Ballou*, opposite Lee Marvin, playing a schoolmarm-turned-outlaw. Elia Kazan invited Fonda to interview for a film he was casting, *Splendor in the Grass*; when he asked if she was ambitious, she clammed up. Forty years later she still fumed at having lost the part to Natalie Wood. "You know what I should have said to Kazan?" she related to a *New Yorker* writer. "Are you kidding? Of course I'm fucking ambitious!"

That ambition took her back to Paris, where the New Wave filmmakers were all the rage, and she again encountered Vadim, who convinced Fonda to star in the steamy sci-fi spoof *Barbarella*. In it Fonda appeared near naked in a latex body suit, fueling men's fantasies around the world but winning few fans who were women.

She started a long, stormy relationship with Vadim, made more difficult by what Fonda later discovered was Vadim's drinking and addiction to gambling, as well as his habit of bringing home call girls to share their bed. She came back to Hollywood, married to Vadim but without him, and began a busy career in film, winning her second Oscar for *Coming Home*, the 1978 film about the challenges facing a disabled Vietnam War vet. Stirred to outrage, like millions, about the war, she became active in the GI protest movement. At one gathering she met and was smitten by Tom Hayden, the outspoken founder of Students for a Democratic Society.

An unlikely headline couple—the glamorous Fonda, the charismatic, rough-hewn Hayden—they toured the country to stoke sentiment against the war, largely in support of the GI protest movement. In 1972 Fonda traveled to North Vietnam to condemn what she believed was the U.S. bombing campaign against the dikes of the Yellow River, whose destruction would have led to widespread starvation. Her broadcasts on Radio Hanoi were viewed with some hostility back home—but nothing like the shock that followed the dissemination of a photo of Fonda smiling atop a Vietcong antiaircraft gun emplacement.

Fonda would lay blame for the photo on circumstances and her own fatigue at the end of a grueling tour. She would later apologize, affirming her support of the American soldiers. But the damage was done, and she was quickly branded "Hanoi Jane."

How startling, then, that a mere two years later the actress—condemned by a rising tide of feminists for her role in *Barbarella*, reviled as a traitor to American men in uniform—would become a publishing phenomenon, topping best-selling charts for her how-to exercise bible, *The Jane Fonda Workout Book*.

Its genesis was Fonda's interest in starting a business that would support Hayden's work on behalf of GIs. Brainstorming, she had even considered an auto repair shop where people would not be ripped off. In the end it was a remark by her stepmother, Shirlee, that sent her down another path. She had fractured her foot in the last week of shooting *The China Syndrome* and needed to get in shape for her next movie, *California Suite*, which required her to appear in a bikini. Shirlee suggested Gilda Marx, and Fonda became a fan. She was raving about the classes, how great they made her feel and how other women loved them, too, when Shirlee said, "You could open a studio, too, you know."

Not long after, Fonda hired Leni Cazden, the main instructor at Gilda's, to help her master the routines in private and dispatched her spy to Century City. Marx was predictably outraged and later contemplated a lawsuit, which an attorney persuaded her to drop, since Gilda had not lost business. "Jane helped me," Marx would admit. "I began the exercise business. She made it world-famous."

The workout itself debuted in Fonda's studio in Beverly Hills and attracted a mob of fellow actors and wannabes. Two years later, in 1982, Scribner's published the first *Workout* book illustrated with photos of Shirlee, an apparent sop to Fonda's stepmother who was miffed that Jane had never credited her with the idea. The book was an instant best seller and was eventually translated into fifty languages. Its reach could be illustrated when, a quarter century later, a young street performer and nightclub dancer in Cali, Colombia, was asked by a gym owner to fill in for an injured aerobics teacher. He agreed but, knowing nothing about aerobics, rushed out and bought a copy of *The Jane Fonda Workout Book*. The young man's name was Alberto Perez, and he would go on to become a multimillionaire as the founder of Zumba.

After the book sold 2 million copies in hardcover, Simon and Schuster threw Fonda a champagne party to toast her success and presented Fonda with a $1.2 million royalty check, the highest royalty check the publisher had ever paid out. She followed it with the *Pregnancy, Birth, and Recovery Workout Book*, which sold another 250,000 copies. Both were ghosted by Fonda's friend Mignon McCarthy.

The best, arguably, was yet to come. That year of the book's publication, 1982, the first of the *Jane Fonda Workout* videos appeared in stores, and it made history. For three years it stayed at the top of the video best-seller list—the first nonmovie to take first spot on the list. It not only made Fonda even more of a fitness icon but also transformed the videotape industry. Previously, most everyone had rented tapes. Fonda's was the first to sell in such numbers. Seventeen million copies later, it remains the biggest-selling home video of all time. "I didn't know what a video *was*," said Fonda. "Nobody knew. You couldn't afford the hardware. The reason it sold so many was there was nothing else out there."

Before you could say, "Feel the burn!" there was an entire look-alike business. Given the state of fitness at the time, videos were an idea waiting to happen. Clubs then were only beginning to appear in urban hubs, malls, and shopping centers. Not everyone had access to a Jazzercise studio—or wanted to get dressed and drive to a gym. It was so much simpler, and cheaper, to roll up the living room rug and plug in a tape. Fonda had a movie star name and best-selling book to trade on, but that did not stop more obscure gym mavens from capitalizing on what she had started. Up in Anchorage, Alaska, a world-class pole vaulter named Gregg Smithey was showcasing his muscle and moves at his Hip Hop Aerobics Club. As a fitness instructor, he could later lay claim to training the state's future governor and vice presidential candidate, Sarah Palin; in 1987 he was a lot more famous as the creator and star of *Buns of Steel*.

The forty-minute routine paid scant heed to aerobics except as a brief warm-up. Instead it was a series of intense lower-body exercises that focused on the butt, legs, and thighs. It was followed in short order by *Abs of Steel* and more in the *Steel* franchise that made Smithey rich, at least briefly. Others had more enduring success.

"Jane Fonda, Raquel Welch, Victoria Principal, Linda Evans are all promoting exercise programs. But I'm not just an actress trying to write an exercise book. My background is fitness. I know what I do. I enjoy it." The speaker was Kathy Smith. It was 1983, and Smith had just been named the new model and spokeswoman for "Babe," the hot Fabergé perfume from Mariel Hemingway. The daughter of an air force pilot, she had grown up in Brazil, Hawaii, and Beverly Hills, an early gymnast and outspoken "tomboy." To promote the "adventurous woman" lifestyle of Babe, she had signed on to skydive, scuba, and river raft. The thirty-one-year-old Smith already had an exercise studio, talked up her *Ultimate Workout* book on television, and trained tennis star Chris Evert Lloyd. Aerobics was in her DNA. "I've always had a hyper kind of energy," she explained. "When I was at college in Hawaii I splashed on the beach oil and sat on the sand like everyone else — for ten minutes. Then I got restless and had to go surf."

"My aspiration," she announced at her Babe promotion, "is to be the Number One fitness person in the country twenty years from now." There's little dispute that she succeeded. She put out dozens of DVDs and books, from her *Feed Muscle, Shrink Fat Diet* to *Moving through Menopause*. She championed exercise for the elderly and sports for girls. She was a fixture on television talk shows. Thirty years after she signed on with Babe, her empire of DVDs, lifestyle products, and fitness equipment had grossed fifty million dollars.

THE SULTAN OF SWEAT

Smith, like many fitness mavens and workout stars, made only oblique reference to the reason most women chose to exercise: weight loss. Even Fonda — especially Fonda, the longtime bulimic — left that motive on the cutting-room floor. It was left to a man to speak the unspoken and tap that huge market, though if one had to cast the ideal man to lead a women's weight-loss crusade, it would likely have been a beach-buff specimen with dreamboat eyes and a rock-hard chin. It would never, in a million years, have been Richard Simmons.

Yet Simmons, for an astonishing forty-plus years, would secure an iconic place in the annals of fitness. He might not be, as his website declaimed, "the nation's most revered fitness expert," but there could be no denying his impact or his longevity as a media personality. His willingness to play the camp clown, dressing up in outrageous outfits or vegetable suits, never detracted from his mission to make Americans proud of their bodies, no matter their shape. He inveighed against dangerous fat and calories, but he also preached acceptance. As one of his skit characters, Reverend Pounds, declared: "Though I waddle through the valley of linguine and clams, I shall fear no evil."

Simmons came to his lifework as a former fattie. A New Orleans native, he grew up in the French Quarter, "where lard was a food group," often made miserable by a "perfect" older brother. To compensate he ate. At age fifteen his weight topped 185 pounds. Graduating from high school, he had ballooned to 268 pounds. He graduated from Florida State University with a degree in art and moved to New York, working as a waiter and for various cosmetics companies. In the early 1970s he settled in Los Angeles. Determined to lose weight, he became a diet fanatic and dropped 112 pounds in two and a half months. He exercised with Gilda Marx and in 1975 opened his own studio, the Anatomy Asylum. Its aim was to entice exercisers who were not already in shape, several of whom appeared with Simmons on the TV show *Real People*.

Soon he was all over television. He was a frequent guest on game shows and had a recurring role as himself during a four-year run on *General Hospital*. He launched a morning exercise show, *The Richard Simmons Show*, which blanketed the country and drew a daily audience of 4.6 million viewers, prompting *People* to call him the "monster of the morning . . . the strongest challenger yet to [Phil] Donahue's daytime dominance." His mix of over-the-top antics and earthy sincerity drew overflow crowds wherever he went and resulted in twenty-five thousand daily letters. Though he never discussed his sexual preferences, he lived alone in the Hollywood Hills with two maids and three Dalmatians and was, most everyone assumed, gay—if not in practice, then certainly in his willingness to act the part. He was, in the words of one academic, a "blend of queer sensibility and shopping mall culture," but he appeared immune to any characterization, even as he feasted on the more outrageous. Endless spoofs did nothing to deter Simmons, who tooled around Beverly Hills in a luxury Mercedes sedan with a "YRUFATT" license plate and a stuffed pig in the passenger seat.

Nobody, not Smith, not Fonda, came close to his output of video cassettes, which numbered close to forty and included *No Ifs, Ands, or Butts*, *Broadway Blast Off*, and the megaselling series *Sweatin' to the Oldies*. He reprised many on DVDs. His *Never-Say-Diet Book* sold six hundred thousand copies.

The year he turned sixty, 2008, was the twentieth anniversary of *Sweatin' to the Oldies*, and Simmons was running around the country to promote it—and himself. A *Chicago Tribune* reporter, covering Simmons's whirlwind tour through the city and suburbs, felt obliged to reveal his secrets—his four-thousand-follicle hair transplant, his closet Catholicism, his canny assumed persona. "The biggest thing you don't know about Simmons," noted the writer, "is that he's in on the joke."

It was only a joke if you didn't take fitness seriously.

Exercise, unlike many sports, was basically a solo activity. It demanded no tryouts and brooked little organization. It required no team uniform and only minimal equipment, especially if the exercise was cardiovascular. In time the sportswear industry would seize on the interest in fitness to sell all manner of specialized clothes. A franchise store such as Sports Authority could boast endless racks devoted to the supposedly unique demands of golf, hiking, tennis. Running shorts were useless for rowing; a cycling top required a wick-proof fiber; no one climbed in cotton. It could be said that each brand's touted line boosted interest in fitness. It could be said that fitness was what propelled the brand. Both statements would be true, and nowhere more so than in the synergistic coupling that wed the athletic shoe to aerobics and running.

Long before Fonda, Sorenson, and Missett, the global market in athletic shoes belonged almost exclusively to Adidas. Based in a tiny Bavarian village of ten thousand people, the company owed its roots to Adi Dassler who, in the waning days of World War I, helped set up a family shoemaking factory in the back of his mother's laundry. With material scavenged from the debris of war—rucksacks, tires, helmets—the sports-minded Adi moved into cleated soccer boots and gym shoes. The product eventually made its way to America, and, in the 1936 Berlin Olympics, Jesse Owens won his four gold medals in black leather Dassler shoes. A family feud erupted after World War II between Adi and his brother Rudi. Neither wanted to cede the Dassler name, so Rudi set up his factory across the town river and called his product Puma; Adi went with Addas, which quickly became Adidas.

For decades the Puma-Adidas rivalry seesawed back and forth, with both companies exploiting soccer championships and Olympics to showcase their shoes. About all they agreed on was the superiority of German shoemaking, and no one paid much attention to competition across the Atlantic. There it was all about the "sneaker," the rubber-soled leisure-time shoe that enjoyed a surge of popularity during the fifties when school dress codes relaxed. The bump in athletic sneakers—endorsed by football star Jim Thorpe and basketball player Chuck Taylor, who lent his name to Converse All Stars—posed little threat in Bavaria, where Germans controlled the sport-shoe market. The battle for the

American market eventually went to Adidas, which topped Puma with its higher-quality shoes and grip on global publicity. In 1964 athletes in Adidas shoes took ninety-nine medals at the Tokyo Olympics—that was what made headline news in the Dasslers' tiny factory town, not two Americans, Phil Knight and Bill Bowerman, who started a company that same year in a place called Oregon.

Bowerman had been Knight's running coach at the University of Oregon. Like Prefontaine, Knight began wearing the footwear inventions Bowerman created to increase time and reduce injury. Unlike his gruff, flamboyant coach, Knight was shy and reserved, so seemingly bland that his college classmates pigeonholed him as an accountant, which is what he became after earning an MBA at Stanford. Few imagined he would go on to build the world's most successful sports company and become a billionaire in the process. "Those who had liked and respected him throughout his first twenty-five years were nonetheless stunned by his success," wrote J. B. Strasser, Nike's first advertising manager and longtime Knight crony. "Mind-boggling" was how Knight's college roommate and fellow track team member Bill Cromwell put it. "He was really a straight shooter. Nothing outstanding. . . . I would not have thought he had this tremendous future ahead of him. That [came] as a great surprise."

Likely it surprised Knight, too. To satisfy a class requirement to create a business idea, he had come up with manufacturing shoes in Japan and selling them in America. Graduating, he took time off to travel and, in the port city of Kobe, Japan, dropped by the Onitsuka Company, which made cheap athletic shoes called Tigers. Asked what company he represented, he made up a name, Blue Ribbon Sports (he had been drinking Pabst Blue Ribbon beer the night before), and had a load of shoes delivered to his parents' garage. He and Bowerman each tossed in five hundred dollars to pay for the product. They peddled the shoes at track meets from the trunk of Knight's car. In 1968 a Bowerman-modified design, "the Cortez," became Tigers' best-selling shoe. Revenues soared to two million dollars, but, after a falling-out over distribution, Blue Ribbon severed ties with Tigers and started manufacture of its own shoe, a latex-and-leather design with the soon-to-be-famous "waffle" sole, which Bowerman had created after tinkering with his wife's waffle iron.

Knight branded the new company Nike after the Greek goddess

Victory; the name had come to Blue Ribbon's first full-time employee, Jeff Johnson, in a dream. The "Swoosh" logo was provided by a local art student, Carolyn Davidson, who submitted an invoice for thirty-five dollars (paid, she received a decade later a still-secret Nike stock certificate). By 1980 Nike controlled half of the market for running shoes in the United States, a booming business after interest in running exploded during the seventies. While Bowerman created new designs, Knight forged savvy alliances with sports celebrities, a strategy that would propel Nike for decades. By the end of 1982, every world record in men's track, from the 800 to the marathon, had been set by athletes wearing Nike's high-performance shoes.

There was only one problem. Focused as it was on elite athletes, Nike failed to notice an even more lucrative demographic: the millions of women who had become aerobics converts and wanted shoes. Nike's corporate counsel, Richard Werschkul, had tried to sound the alarm. He had been drinking in a Portland bar one night when a group of young people came in, sweaty and red-faced. As recounted in *Swoosh*, Nike's unofficial history: "He assumed they had been playing a game of pick-up basketball or volleyball, but he was wrong. They had just come from an aerobics class. On their feet were soft white leather athletic shoes Werschkul had never seen before. After talking to them for an hour, Werschkul phoned Knight. "'Phil,' he said, 'the future is aerobics. Reebok is what's happening. We need aerobic shoes.' Werschkul got the distinct impression that Knight thought either he'd had too much beer, or that he was crazy."

The upstart Reebok had seemed to come out of nowhere, though not to anyone who had seen 1981's Oscar-winning Best Picture, *Chariots of Fire*. The film was the thrilling tale of the 1924 British Olympic track team that pulled off its improbable triumph in clunky hand-sewn shoes by J. W. Foster & Sons. More than a half century later, founder Joe Foster's grandsons had changed the name to Reebok, after the gazelle speedster, but were having limited success. It was not until a thirty-five-year-old Reebok salesman, Paul Fireman, bought the exclusive rights to distribute in North America that the company's fortunes changed. Fireman felt that Nike was overemphasizing the tech aspect of shoes and ignoring the women's casual business, and he marketed Reebok's first aerobic shoe, the Freestyle, with the tagline "Simple Elegance."

Women loved the narrow, flattering fit and soft leather-upper material; the shoes were lighter than Nike's clunky running shoes, almost like slippers. "Ballet shoes that were sneakers!" one trainer called them. In fact, the design was something of an accident. Reebok had its shoes manufactured in China, where it shipped the pattern. When the shoes came back, Reebok was horrified to see they had been made from glove, not shoe, leather. With the shipment a total loss, the shoes were tossed in big buckets—and sold out instantly.

Nike would continue to thrive with new products and aggressive marketing. It tapped big-name sports figures, recruiting the likes of Tiger Woods and Michael Jordan, whose Air Jordan would prove the most successful athlete endorsement in history, selling more than $100 million in a single year. It expanded into apparel, ever more desirable as health clubs boomed in the eighties; and women, in particular, found gyms a new showcase to exhibit their fashion style and shape. It promoted fitness as a fun, all-encompassing lifestyle, and its NikeTown retail stores were an attempt to move the habit of exercise from the athletic field and cardio floor into the rialto, to give it the flash of entertainment, combining, as the company promised, "the fun and excitement of FAO Schwartz, the Smithsonian Institution and Disneyland."

But the pesky Reebok grew into a major threat, and in 1985 its sales reached $307 million, ten times what they had been just three years before. Fireman appeared on magazine covers as the highest-paid executive in America, thanks to a lucrative incentive plan. Aerobics, however, had begun to reach the outer limit of growth, in part a victim of its own popularity. As more instructors were drawn to the field, the more they devised complex routines to stand out from the competition. The average client simply could not keep up and lost interest, and the numbers began to flatline and then tail off. To pick up the slack, the big athletic shoe companies—Nike, Reebok, and Converse—tried to convince consumers that walking was every bit as good an exercise as aerobics.

In a 1987 *Chicago Tribune* article, "Athletic Shoe Boom Slows to a Fast Walk," the well-known miler Marty Liquori confirmed the update from the chain of sporting-goods stores he had founded. "After being talked about by manufacturers for several years, walking is finally being talked about by consumers."

Fireman was more cautious. "Walking is like water. It's free. The hardest thing to sell somebody is something that's free," he said, then quickly added, "Nobody thought you could sell water, but then along came Perrier, which proved the right kind of water costs money."

At Avia, the shoe company, spokeswoman Kellee Harris offered this bit of optimism: "In the past, people have looked at walking as being a geriatric activity. But we're finding there's a whole new generation out there into walking. People are walking in malls and around their neighborhoods. There are walking classes and walking clubs all over the country. We think they are going to be the next singles clubs."

Walking clubs were not the next singles clubs. An initial surge in sales of so-called walking shoes—among women; men, if they walked, did so in basketball shoes—soon faded. Nike reverted to what it did best: sports. Reebok would likely have slipped further into second-place status had not Fireman gotten wind of a new fitness craze that had started in Atlanta, Georgia. Apparently, classes there were packed with women who climbed up and down on a plastic step to music. The woman who ran the classes had worked up elaborate routines. Fireman's vice president of business development, Angel Martinez, said she was spunky and bright and attractive. He was very excited. He was flying her to Los Angeles to give a demonstration.

The woman with the step was Gin Miller. Born in Connecticut, an avid athlete, she had taken up gymnastics in high school and kept at it at Georgia Tech but eventually switched to a career in fitness because, as she explained, "it seemed the thing that gymnasts did when they got too old. Aerobics was becoming a huge cult then. In those days if you were a gymnast or dancer, you naturally became an aerobics instructor."

Graduating, she started coaching kids' gymnastics and ran conditioning classes for the parents. She stayed sharp competing in contests—dance aerobics or jazz dance—and always won top prize. Her own aerobics classes were filled to the walls, and she was teaching twenty a week—until she twisted her knee.

The conditioning coach at Georgia Tech recommended she climb up and down on a milk crate to get her mobility back. Miller tried it, found it boring, and switched to her porch steps at home. To motivate herself, she went inside and put music on the stereo, threw open the window, and began marching up and down the porch. She devised a foot-square bench and tried it out at the aerobics studio where she was teaching classes again. She partnered with the owners of a health club, the Sports Life, and launched the Step Company, which built brightly colored plastic steps. Confident she was on to something, she made a film of her routines and sent it to the Patent Office. She had the film with her when she met Martinez and Fireman in Los Angeles. "That's what protected me when I took it to Reebok. They completely overhauled it, and it became the world's next great fitness craze," she said with a laugh.

It was the perfect exercise: low impact, high intensity; it burned as many calories as running at 7.2 miles an hour. The music made it even more compelling: "With a percussive backbeat, it's very tribal; it has a ritualistic marching movement," Miller explained. Add weights, and you worked the upper body. "If you can use all four limbs and the trunk in a movement pattern, anyone in fitness will tell you—you've got it made."

Reebok had a ready-made test group. Selling its Freestyle shoe, it had tucked a slip of paper inside offering a discount to any trainer. Using that database, Miller and Reebok sent off six hundred brochures—and got an enthusiastic response to almost every one. The program was branded Step Reebok, launching a thirteen-year relationship between Reebok and Miller. In time Miller would travel worldwide to set up trainings in sixty-seven countries and put out seven top-selling videos and DVDs. In 1991 she was named "Instructor of the Year" by the International Dance Exercise Association (IDEA), the preeminent organization for group-exercise professionals. Step aerobics grew so popular that, in 1994, the company set up Reebok University in Indianapolis to coordinate the hundreds of "master trainers" across the United States.

"What took it over the edge, what made it so unique," said Miller, "beyond all the stuff in the press release, was everyone had their own space. With regular aerobics, people were running into each other. With step you had your own five-by-four square. Nobody touched your stuff. You had a classroom, with all the social benefits, but you also had your own space. That's what worked so well."

Reebok tried to capitalize on its step success with any number of programs in the 1990s, most of which were returned to the branding book. Few, for instance, will remember "Slide Reebok," which the company aggressively hyped to clubs as another Next Big Thing, and Reebok University closed up shop in 1998. Miller, as was her wont, kept on going. She opened her own club in Atlanta in the spring of 2012, more an exercise evangelist than ever. "What makes fitness great? It's fun. Anybody can do it. It's not gender specific. And it gets the job done. It alleviates stress and depression and disease — it does everything to make a person happier. What takes it over the edge," she continued, "is it's social. There's so much disconnectivity now. But we need to have *human* connections; really, we're hungry for the human touch. Instead, all we touch is our phones or iPods or computers. People are finally starting to realize, 'Ugh, it's wearing me out!'"

CHAPTER 6

The Buff Culture, 1970s–1990s

The Weiders build an empire; the Austrian Oak takes charge; star power adds muscle to Hollywood; women are strong, too

THE BARONS OF BODYBUILDING

Running, as an activity and sport, continued its appeal to Americans who believed a cardio workout was essential to fitness. It did not make true believers of everyone. The typical ectomorph runner's body was diametrically opposite from what many deemed the true benchmark of fitness: superior muscle strength. To be sure, there had been other standards. The fitness test for youth employed by Kraus and Prudden measured flexibility (ability to touch one's toes) and modest strength (leg lifts, push-ups). But neither suppleness nor a healthy heart deflected a segment of the population from a more consuming goal: the ability to lift impressive piles of iron, or look able to do so. Whether a sign of virility, the manifest reward of hard work, or a badge of self-confidence, a buff body delivered untold benefits. No one in the modern era did more to promote that pursuit than two brothers: Joe Weider and Ben Weider.

Both were big fans of bodybuilding and developed impressive physiques, especially Joe, though neither competed in contests. Together, they founded the International Federation of Bodybuilders (IFBB) as well as the Mr. Olympia and Ms. Olympia contests. What made them famous and rich, first and foremost, was their magazine publishing empire, which came to include *Muscle and Fitness*, *Flex*, *Men's Fitness*, and *Shape*, spawning a hugely profitable line of supplements, equipment, books, and training manuals. Their growing prominence ignited the sport's infamous bitch-slapping circus—the decades-long feud with archrival and York Barbell patriarch Bob Hoffman. Joe would also lay claim to transforming a blubbery bodybuilder from Austria into the greatest muscled specimen since Charles Atlas.

Their saga began in a seedy neighborhood of Montreal, Canada, the sons of a Polish immigrant father who toiled for nickels and dimes in a garment factory. It was a hardscrabble life. The Weiders' first son died at two months of undetermined causes; their second was the victim of childhood rheumatic fever and would succumb to its complications at age thirty. Joe and younger brother Ben looked headed for an equally grim fate, both scrawny and bullied by neighborhood toughs. Worse, they had the added stigma of being Jewish. Both dropped out of school, Joe at age ten to take a job hauling groceries in a wagon. Far from discouraging him, the routine apparently fueled his interior fantasies, turning him into a "creative thinker" who was soon a regular at the local library. "I was frightened of being ignorant and left behind," he wrote in *Brothers of Iron*, the joint autobiography he coauthored with Ben, "so I studied the writings of philosophers and great thinkers—Nietzsche, Freud, Schopenhauer, Marx, and so on. . . . I examined everything, testing it with my own reason and writing out commentaries and criticism that deepened my understanding and also protected my independence. I remember coming to a chapter written by Schopenhauer where he asked, 'What is an intelligent man?' He said it had nothing to do with years of university study and professorships and that sort of thing."

When he was not reading Schopenhauer, and freed from wasted time in school, he got interested in weight lifting. In his early teens he stumbled on a photograph of a young John Grimek in the magazine *Strength*. Unable to afford a real barbell set, he scouted a railway graveyard and got an attendant to weld two flywheels to a rusty iron shaft. Now there was no stopping him. He lifted, he trained, he got neighboring weight lifter George F. Jowett to sell a barbell set on a layaway plan. At the age of seventeen, and with a scant seven dollars in his pocket, he started his own magazine, what would become *Your Physique*, by lifting subscribers' names from a "Pen Pal" section in Bob Hoffman's *Strength and Health*. It was a crude twelve-page mimeographed newsletter that Joe typed with two fingers on a rented typewriter. He quit his job as a short-order cook and hired a professional printer for issue number 2. To subsidize costs he tapped a local foundry to build barbells and dumbbells, using the magazine to sell them. Essentially, the magazine became a mail-order catalog for Weider-brand products, "but with excellent editorial content and pictures," Weider added.

The formula worked wonders, and within years he relocated across the border, first to Jersey City, then to a warehouse in Brooklyn, which became the seat of his publishing business. He hooked up with a major distributor, American News. He changed the name of *Your Physique* — "too French-sounding and soft for U.S. readers" — to *Muscle Builder* and began branching out. At a time when Hugh Hefner was raking in millions with bare-breasted women and the material delights that awaited in dens and bedrooms, Weider tapped the more active testosterone market with magazines on boxing and wrestling, then *Inside Baseball* and *Inside Sports*. Like Hefner, he had a visceral feel for magazines and what would sell and, urged on by American News, aped *Playboy* with *Jem* and *Monsieur*. He expanded into pulps with action-adventure titles like *Animal Life* and *Safari*. With misgivings he also published *Adonis* and *Body Beautiful* and filled them with pictures of muscled gods and not much clothing. "They became an embarrassment I didn't need," he would later write. "The magazines, which were actually pretty tasteful, naturally sold big to gays and gave Bob Hoffman a new excuse to smear me."

The feud with Hoffman was a pitched playground battle — "the longest craziest pissing match in the history of magazine publishing, also in organized sports," Weider would characterize it, and that was no exaggeration. Though claiming to be above it, Weider referred to the feud repeatedly in *Brothers of Iron*, mostly to settle scores with Hoffman or to denounce the smarmy attacks of his enemy. "Hoffman once called me a kike — in print!" he fumed. "Here's the actual quote from *Strength & Health*. 'Apparently you can take a kike out of the slums, but you can never take the slums out of the kike.'"

Certainly, Hoffman had much to fear from the upstart publishing rival who would eventually eclipse him. As the Weiders expanded their business and Hoffman fought to solidify the insider's edge, they clashed repeatedly in almost every fitness precinct. Weider got scientists and doctors to sign on as magazine consultants, among them Dr. Frederick Tilney, Hoffman's big gun at *Strength and Health* (the same Tilney who suggested Charles Atlas launch a mail-order business). Weider, once he had recruited him, called Tilney "the most forceful, dynamic, and inspiring lecturer on 'The Science of Healthful Living in the world!'"

Hyperbole was never a Weider problem; nor apparently was truth in advertising. To rival Hoffman's claim to science, he started the "Weider Research Clinic" at his headquarters in Union City, New Jersey, though one of his own scientist-consultants admitted "there was no clinic as such." In 1966 when Mr. America, Bob Gajda, visited Weider's offices, he found that the door with the sign "Research Clinic" led to a broom closet.

One of their fiercest battles focused on selling equipment and featured a side skirmish that was pure Keystone Cops comedy. As the Weiders grew their barbell manufacturing business, it became clear they needed a high-profile spokesman to endorse the product. The obvious choice was John Grimek – but Grimek was firmly in the York camp – so Weider tapped a young but extremely muscular bodybuilder, Dan Lurie, the runner-up in three successive Mr. America contests, 1942–44. In each Lurie had won the "Most Muscular" award.

To endorse his barbells, Weider put Lurie in *Your Physique* and featured him on the magazine's cover, and the two men became friends as well as business partners. Shipping costs and import taxes made it prohibitive for Weider to ship weight sets from Canada, so they established the Dan Lurie Barbell Company in the basement of Lurie's parents' home in Brooklyn, enabling Weider to sell barbells to American readers of *Your Physique*. All apparently went smoothly – Weider even stayed at Lurie's parents' home when in New York – until 1945 when Lurie, now a gym owner and pleased with his growing prominence, saw fit to challenge Grimek for the title of "Most Muscular Man in the World." The motive stemmed less from vanity than injustice: Lurie had been barred from competing in the 1946 Mr. America because he had appeared in ads in *Your Physique*. The Mr. America contests were run by the American Athletic Union, which Bob Hoffman controlled – yet Grimek, who appeared in York barbell ads, was deemed an amateur and allowed to compete. It was so unfair. Obviously, the fix was in.

A flurry of letters, charges, and countercharges ensued – most between Lurie and Grimek – with not a few accusing Weider of orchestrating the entire affair to get publicity. Weider flatly denied involvement, and his howl of outrage, expressed forty years later in *Brothers of Iron*, said much about the impossibly tangled battle for the muscle market:

> Give me a break! Never, ever, would I do such a thing: Grimek was my idol. My writers praised him to the skies, and I had just put him on the cover. The way it really happened, Lurie put his challenge into an issue just closing while I was out of town. I came home, saw the challenge, and had a fit, but it was too late to pull the thing out of the magazine. This killed me—and it still kills me—because right then Grimek wanted to come work with me. He told me he was sick of working for Hoffman. But then that stupid challenge spoiled everything. No way would Grimek cross over to the Weider camp if Lurie was part of it. . . . It kills me, it really does. Think about the opportunity missed—Joe Weider and John Grimek, as a team!

The showdown never happened—not exactly. The contest was held in Philadelphia in May 1946 and was won by Grimek. The "Most Muscular Man" portion of the evening turned into an amusing fiasco when Lurie climbed from the audience while Hoffman shouted, "Get the hell off the stage," then competed, in borrowed posing trunks, against a professional wrestler, Walter "the Golden Superman" Podolak, and a fabled but aging bodybuilder, the forty-four-year-old Sig Klein, who had great abdominals but no leg muscles. The judges awarded Lurie second (Klein won)—a verdict greeted with boos and thrown chairs and did nothing to resolve any issues with Grimek, nor did it ease tensions between Lurie and Weider.

The following year, 1947, Weider sued his business partner, claiming Lurie was hiding profits and selling Weider products with a "Dan Lurie Barbell Company" stamp. When process servers failed to find Lurie with legal papers, Weider insisted on accompanying a server to Lurie's gym and chased his onetime friend into a toilet, where Lurie locked himself in. When Lurie tried to bolt free, Weider boasted, "[I] threw a headlock on him and twisted him around and made him take the papers like a gentleman." "That guy," Weider would write, "was like gum on my shoe."

Lurie survived the headlock and busted relations with Weider and went on to achieve considerable success. He hosted big-name bodybuilding contests; published a magazine, *Muscle Training Illustrated*; and became a phenomenon on the 1950s CBS show *The Big Top Circus Show*, appearing as "Sealtest Dan, the Muscle Man." His feats of strength included 1,665 push-ups done in ninety minutes. As his fame waned he attempted to hitch his name to a far bigger star: Steve Reeves. After his last *Hercules* and a few ensuing flops, Reeves had disappeared from view, retiring to a home in the Alps. It was there that Lurie tracked him down and launched a campaign to restore Hercules to his former glory — or at least a new starring role in movies. Ultimately, it all fizzled, though Lurie did succeed in having Reeves's name revived with a succession of plaques and awards, including Lurie's own "Hall of Fame" award.

Why did Reeves — wealthy and comfortable — succumb to Lurie's self-serving campaign to put him back on display? "He probably felt a sense of nostalgia for his bodybuilding roots," speculated *Iron Game* historian John Fair, "and a desire to repay his fans for their generosity over the years. He may also have had a little too much time on his hands."

Lurie, meanwhile, never abandoned efforts to keep his own name in the headlines, and he finally got his wish. In 1984 he sent a letter to the White House, hoping to present President Ronald Reagan with a "Most Fit President of All Time" plaque and, to his surprise, was invited to the Oval Office, where Reagan challenged him to an arm-wrestling contest. A photograph of the event (which Reagan won — twice) appeared on the front page of the *New York Times*.

Weider's legacy is on more solid footing, though his brother Ben gets most credit for founding the International Federation of Bodybuilders. At the time of the Lurie-Grimek flap, the contretemps over amateur status and who sanctioned which contest was becoming a major issue in the world of bodybuilding. The AAU, the leading amateur sports governing body, dated back to 1888 and was firmly in control of amateur weight lifting. It also had a working relationship with the International Olympic Committee. Hoffman, the patriarch of U.S. weight lifting, maintained a stranglehold on the sport in AAU events (not a few have suggested he rigged contests to favor York regulars). In 1939 the AAU began incorporating Mr. America contests into weight-lifting events, and Hoffman, never a fan of physique-type posing, used his influence to ban numerous bodybuilders, several of whom arranged separate professional venues. The conflict reached a boiling point with the 1946 Mr. Canada competition. When the Hoffman-controlled AAU withdrew its sanction at the last minute, the furious Weiders started their own organization: the IFBB.

Though the IFBB would eventually emerge as the sport's reigning sanctioning body — it now runs events in more than 170 countries — it

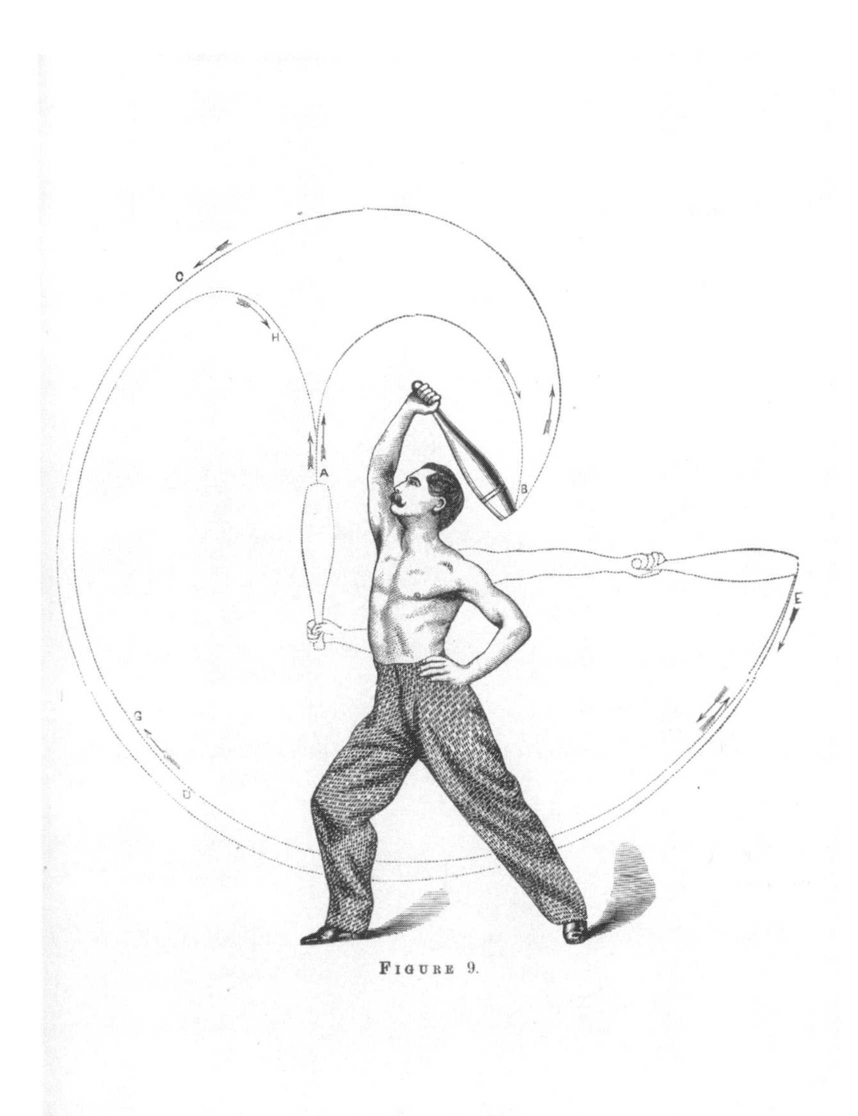

1. S. D. Kehoe's 1866 book, *The Indian Club Exercises*, was hugely popular during the Athletic Revival and the heyday of muscular Christianity. The clubs were favored by early sports teams and were big at churches, which organized "swing club socials." Courtesy of The Strong, Rochester, New York.

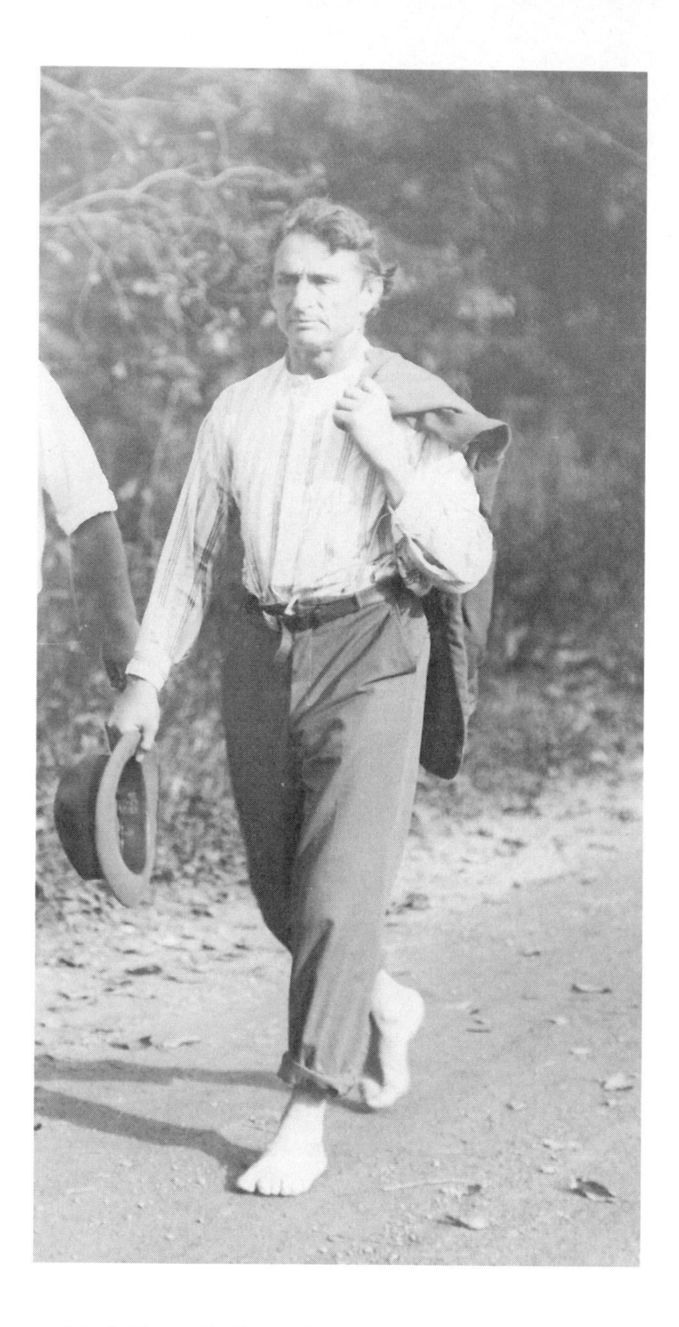

2. Bernarr Macfadden walked six miles to work barefoot. The self-proclaimed "father of physical culture" was especially proud of his hair, displayed on an early cover of his influential magazine along with the motto, "Weakness Is a Crime. Don't Be a Criminal." Courtesy of the Stark Center/University of Texas.

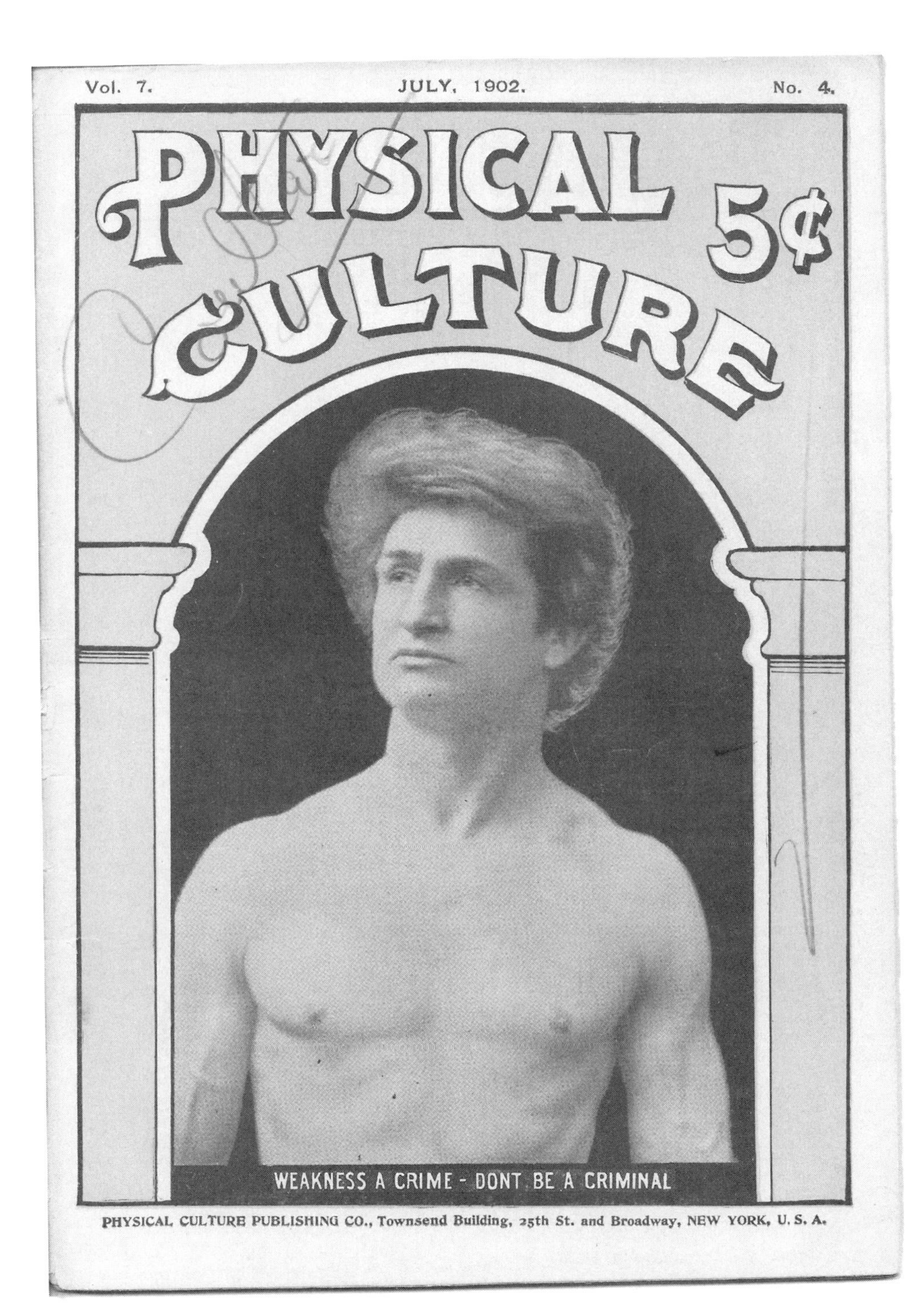
Vol. 7.
JULY, 1902.
No. 4.
PHYSICAL CULTURE
5¢
WEAKNESS A CRIME - DONT BE A CRIMINAL
PHYSICAL CULTURE PUBLISHING CO., Townsend Building, 25th St. and Broadway, NEW YORK, U. S. A.

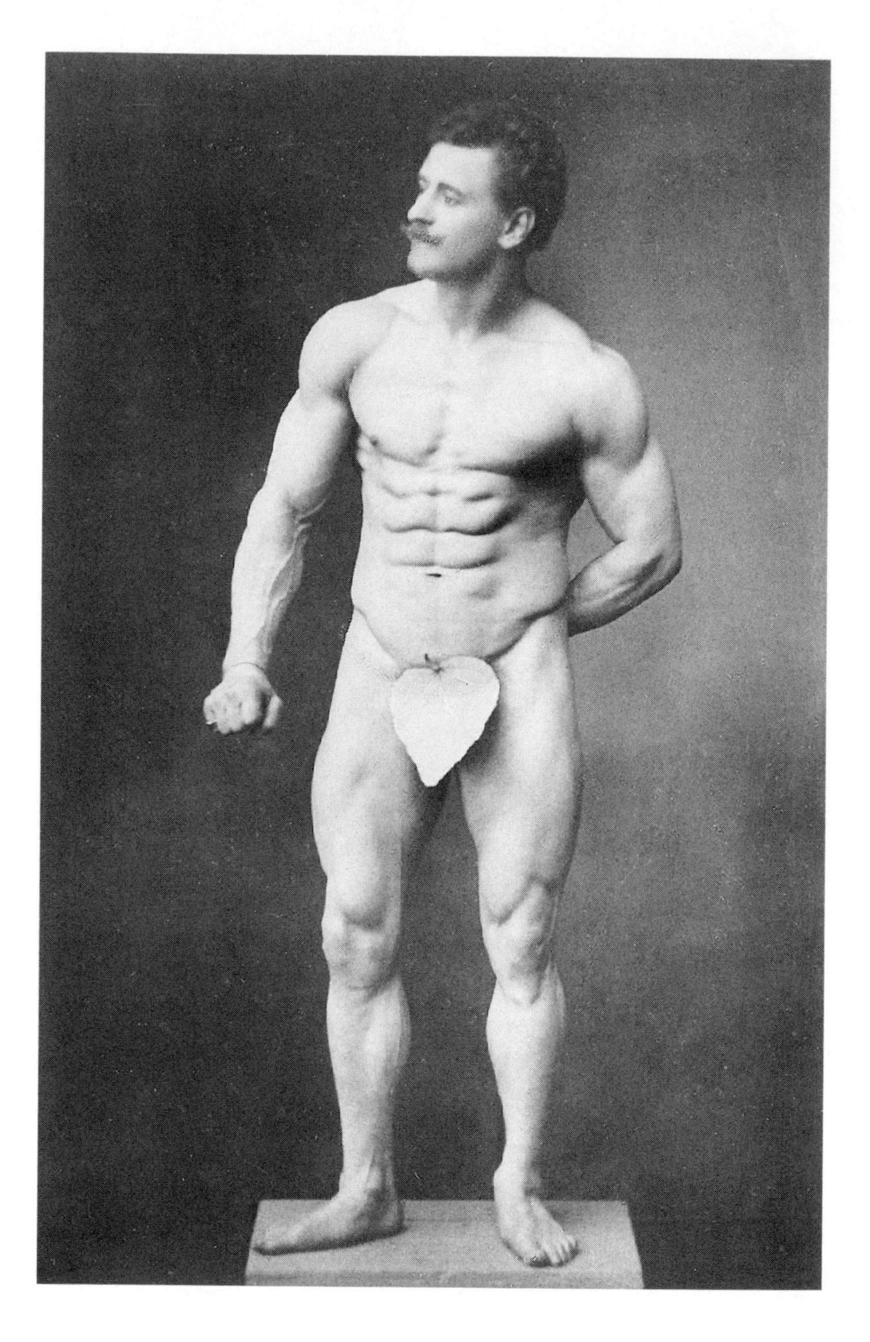

3. Eugen Sandow, the fitness pioneer and vaudeville strongman, caused a sensation during turn-of-the-century U.S. tours promoted by impresario Florenz Ziegfeld. Women who paid for a backstage feel of his biceps were known to faint. Courtesy of David Chapman.

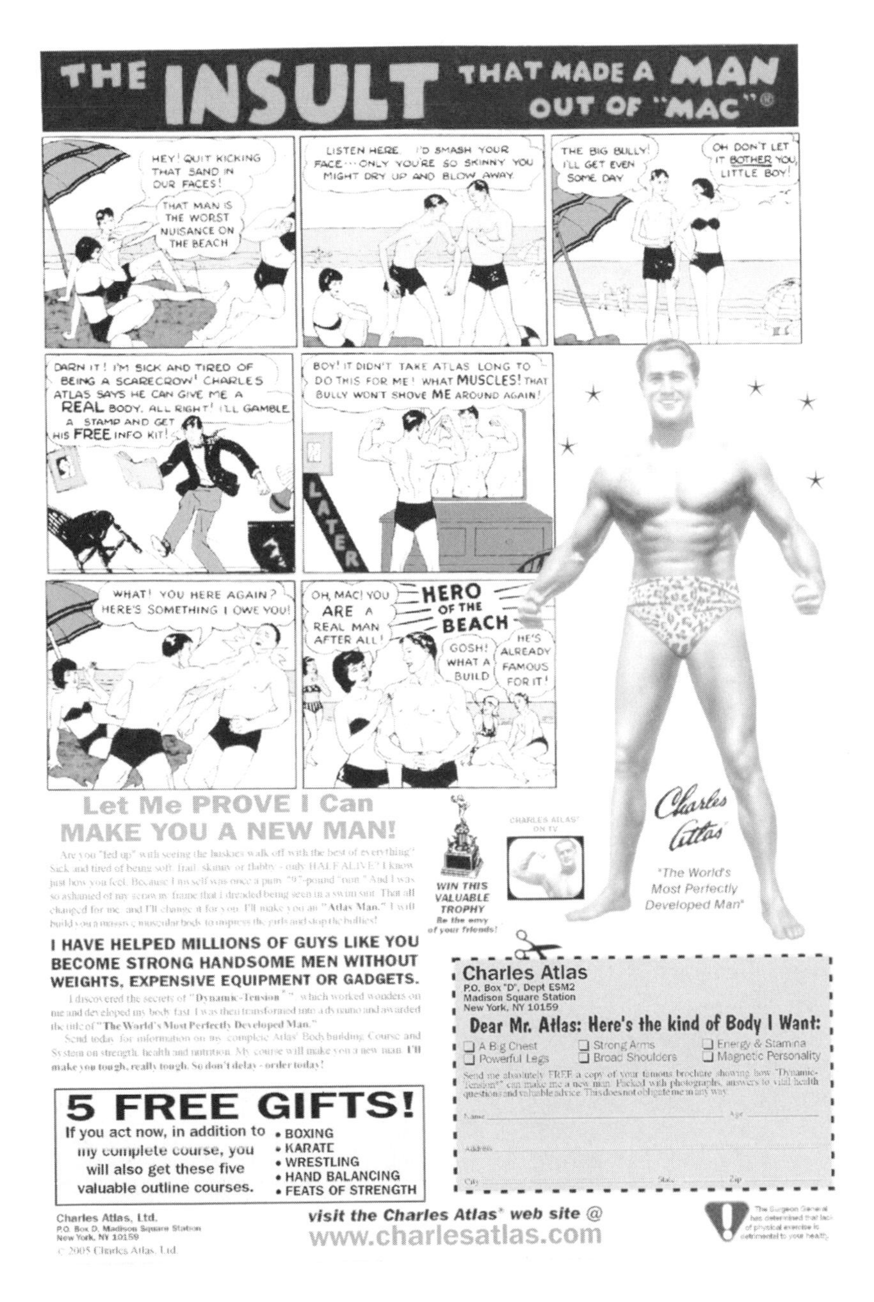

4. Charles Atlas in his most famous ad, which promised ninety-seven-pound weaklings a new body and outlook on life if they bought his system of Dynamic Tension. Seventy years later the company was still in business. "Charles Atlas®." "The Insult That Made A Man Out of Mac®" under license from Charles Atlas, Ltd., PO Box "D", Madison Square Station, New York NY 10159 (www.CharlesAtlas.com).

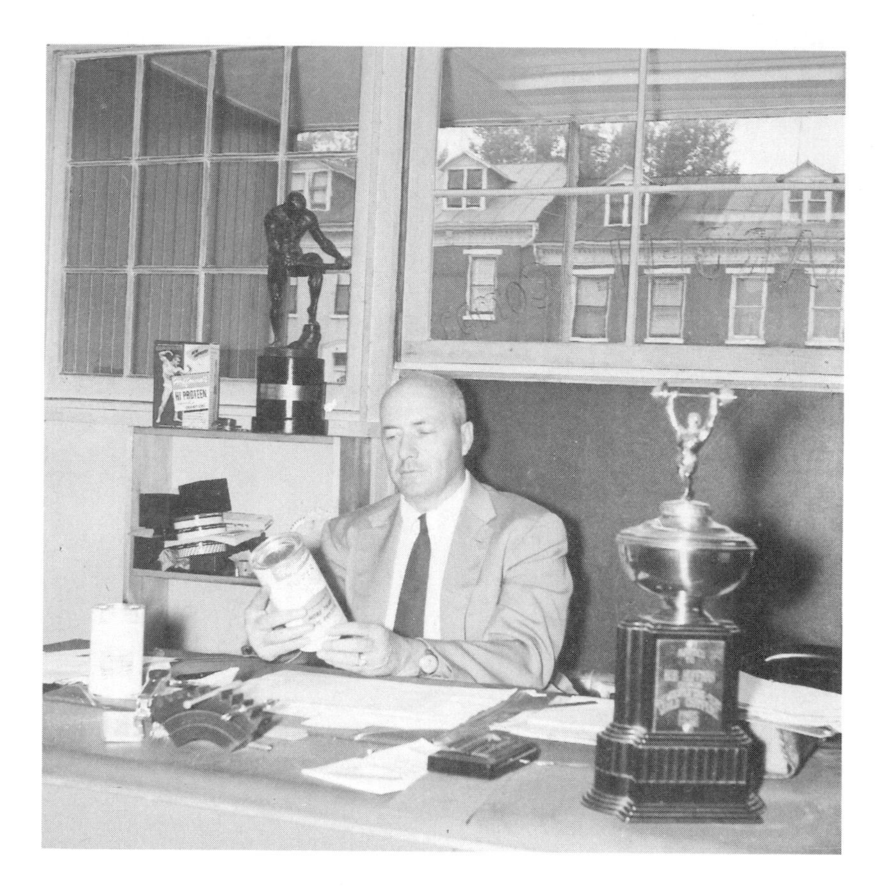

5. Bob Hoffman turned his Pennsylvania oil-burner factory into the world's barbell capital and a mecca for weight lifters. The publisher of *Strength and Health*, he pumped up his acolytes with steroids and profits with his canned protein powder. Courtesy of John Fair.

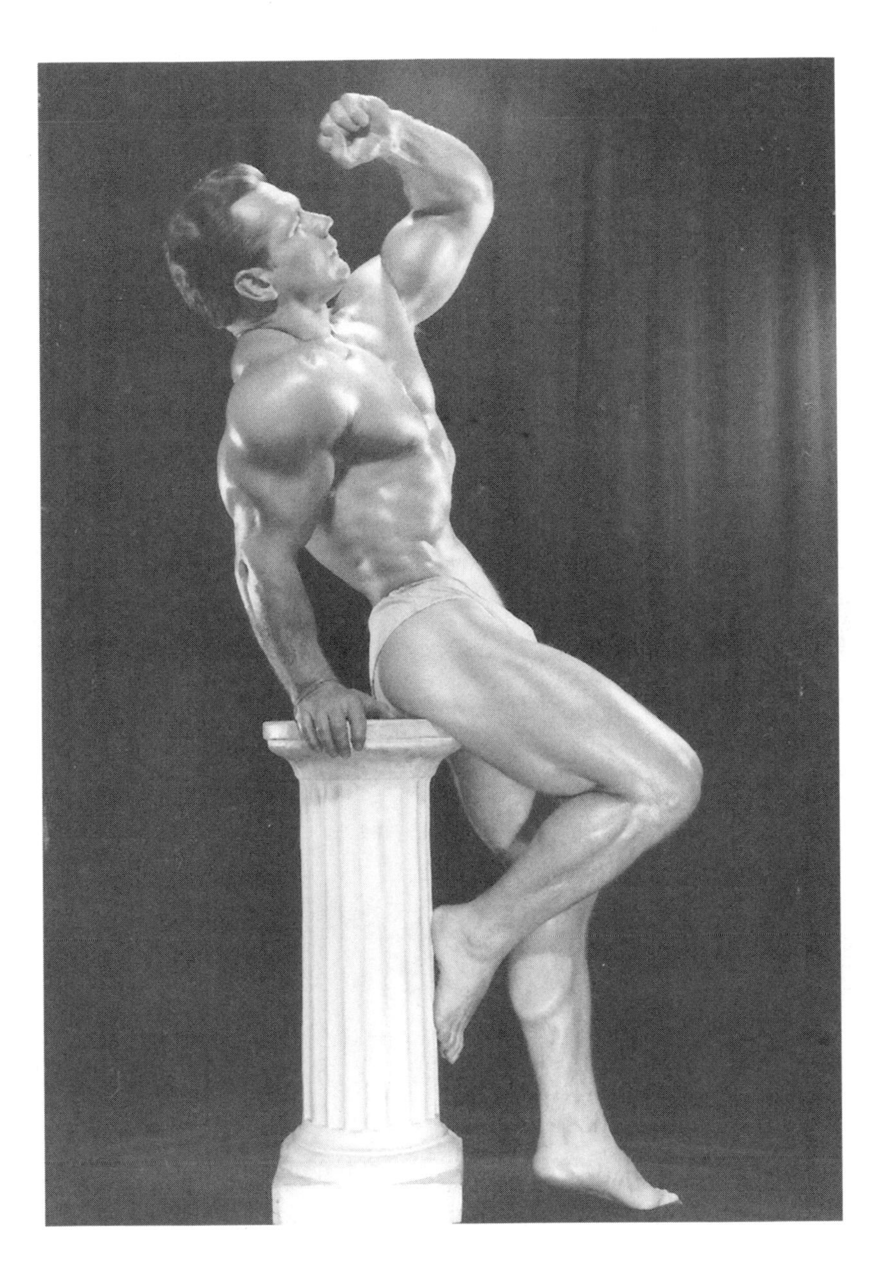

6. John Grimek, a legend in Hoffman's strongman stable, was considered by many the greatest of physique stars for his athleticism and musculature. He so dominated his first two Mr. America contests that the AAU ruled no winner could compete twice. Courtesy of John Fair.

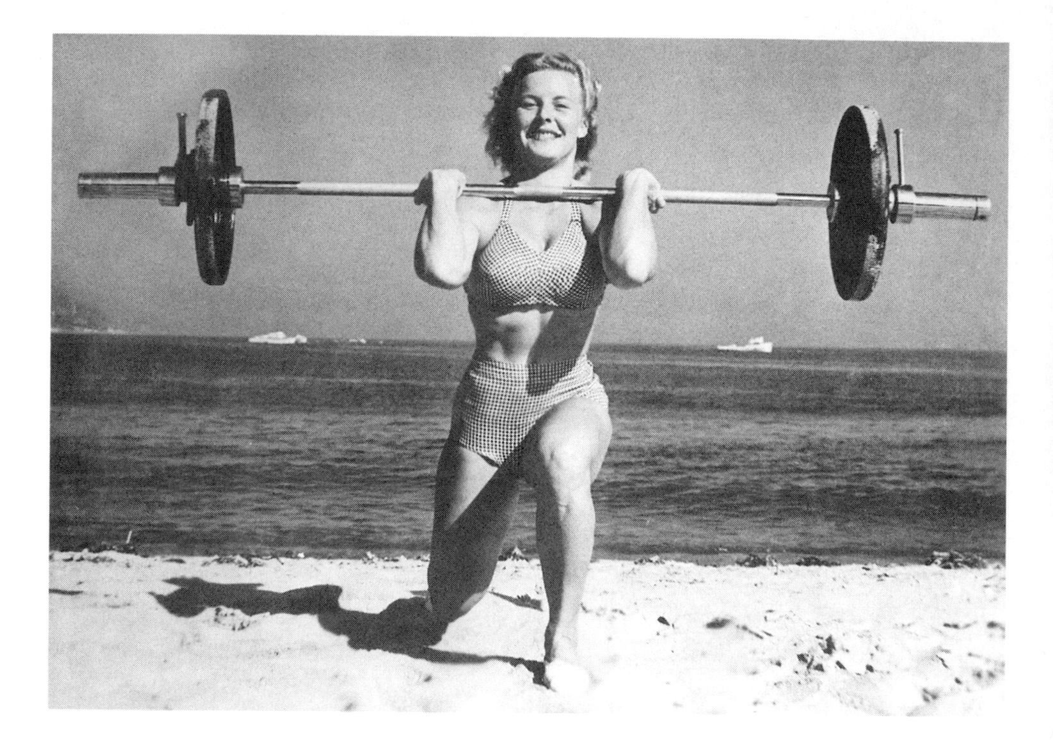

7. (*Above*) Pudgy Stockton, the queen of Santa Monica, was proof that women could build muscle without losing their feminine appeal. She wrote a fitness column called "Barbelles," starred in newsreels, and was featured on forty-two magazine covers. Courtesy of David Chapman.

8. (*Right*) In the forties Muscle Beach was the Santa Monica playground where gymnasts, athletes, and bodybuilders celebrated their strength and feats to cheering crowds. Women played a big part in the show. Courtesy of the Stark Center/University of Texas. Permission granted from Laura Stockton.

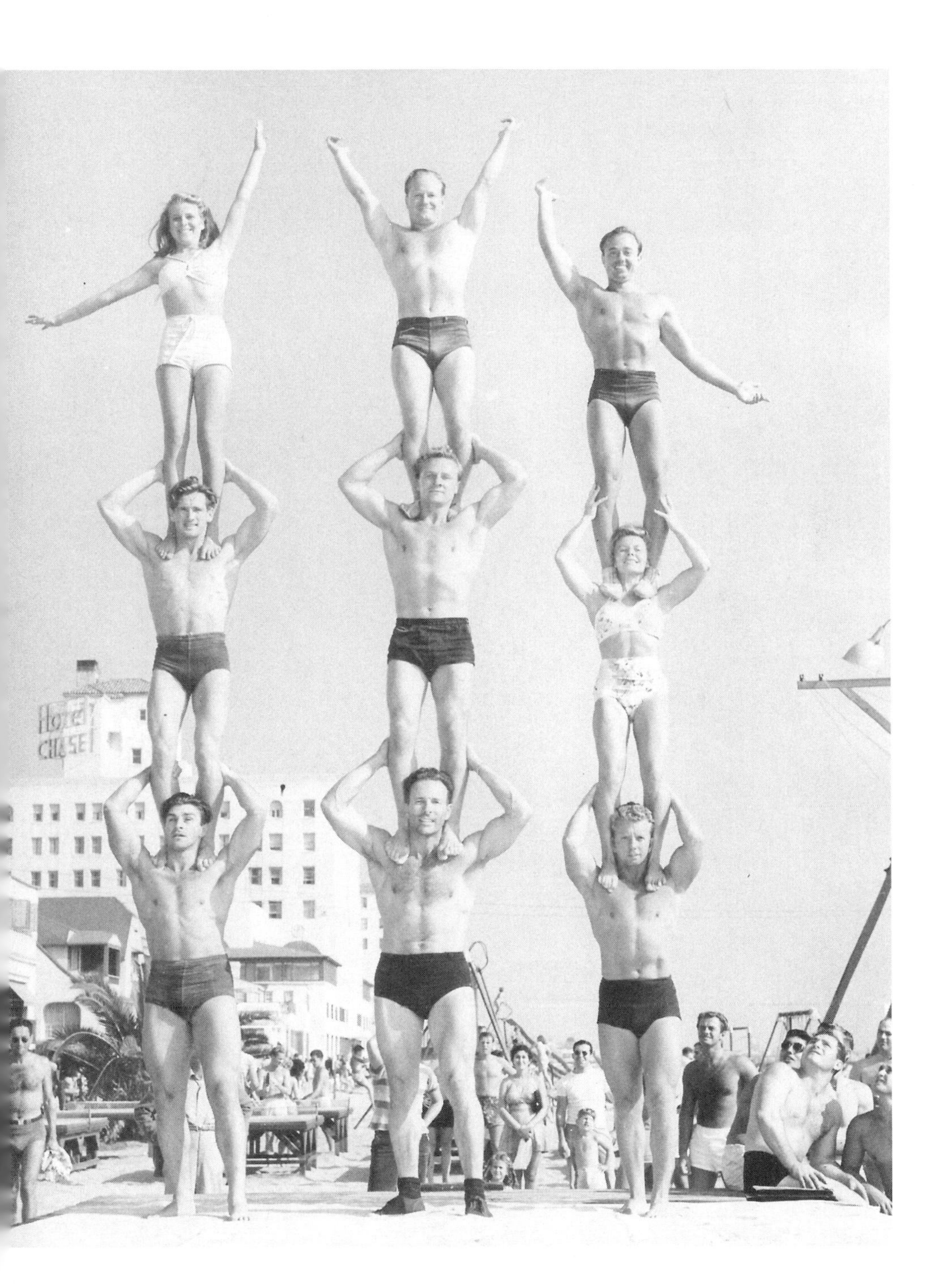
Hotel
CHASE

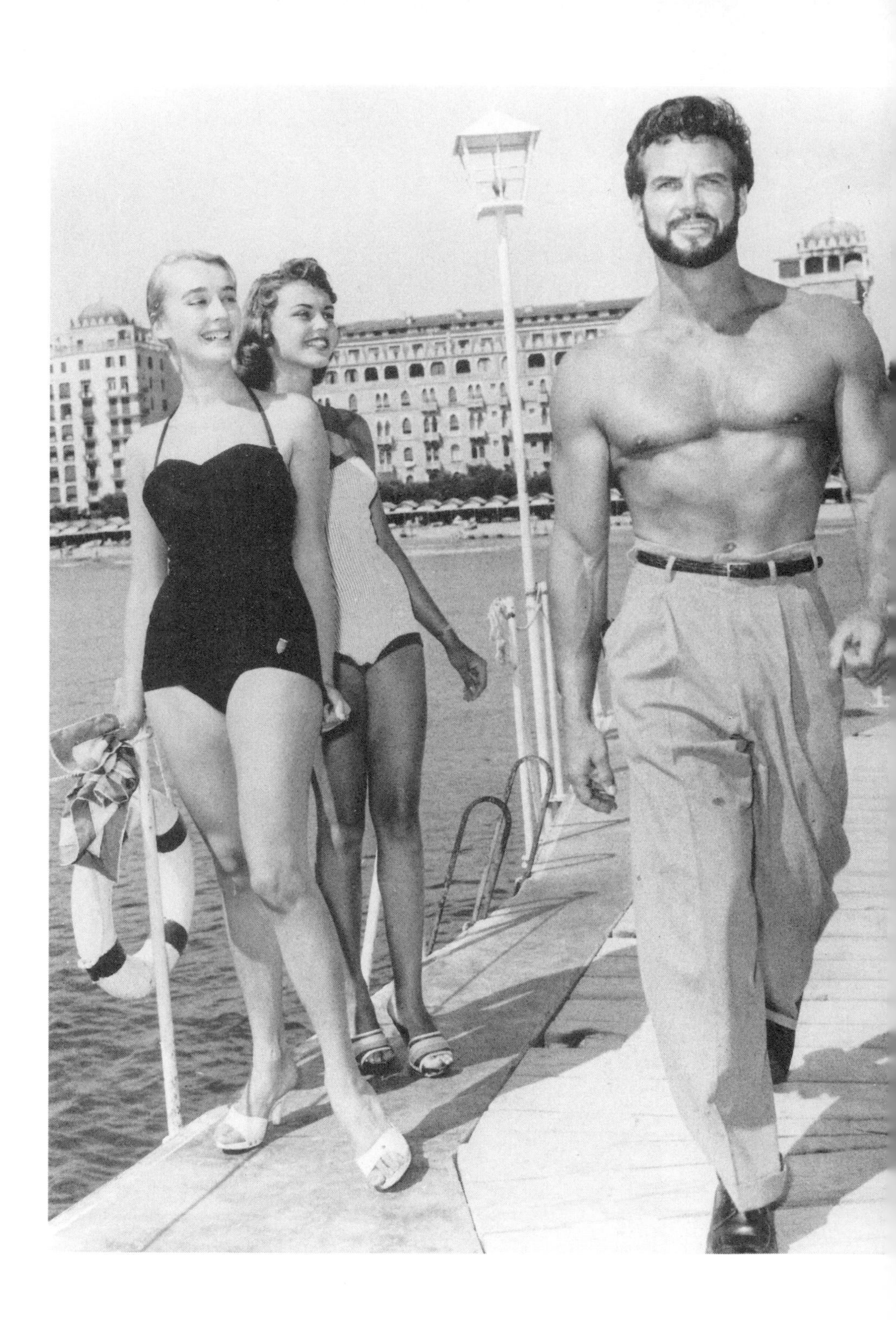

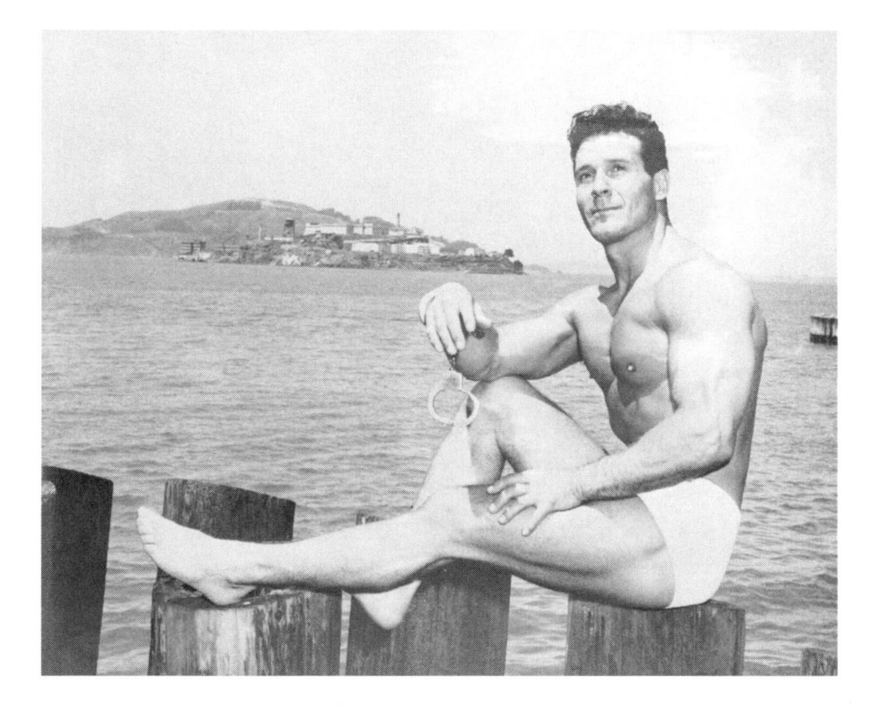

9. (*Left*) The most famous alumnus of Muscle Beach, Steve Reeves, had startling good looks and a chest that stopped traffic. No one cared that his sword-and-sandals epics were dubbed. Courtesy of the Stark Center/University of Texas.

10. (*Above*) Jack LaLanne, the cornball star of fifties television, enchanted the housewives of America in tights and ballet slippers. A serious bodybuilder, he was equally renowned for his birthday stunts such as his manacled swim across San Francisco Bay from Alcatraz. © Bettmann/CORBIS.

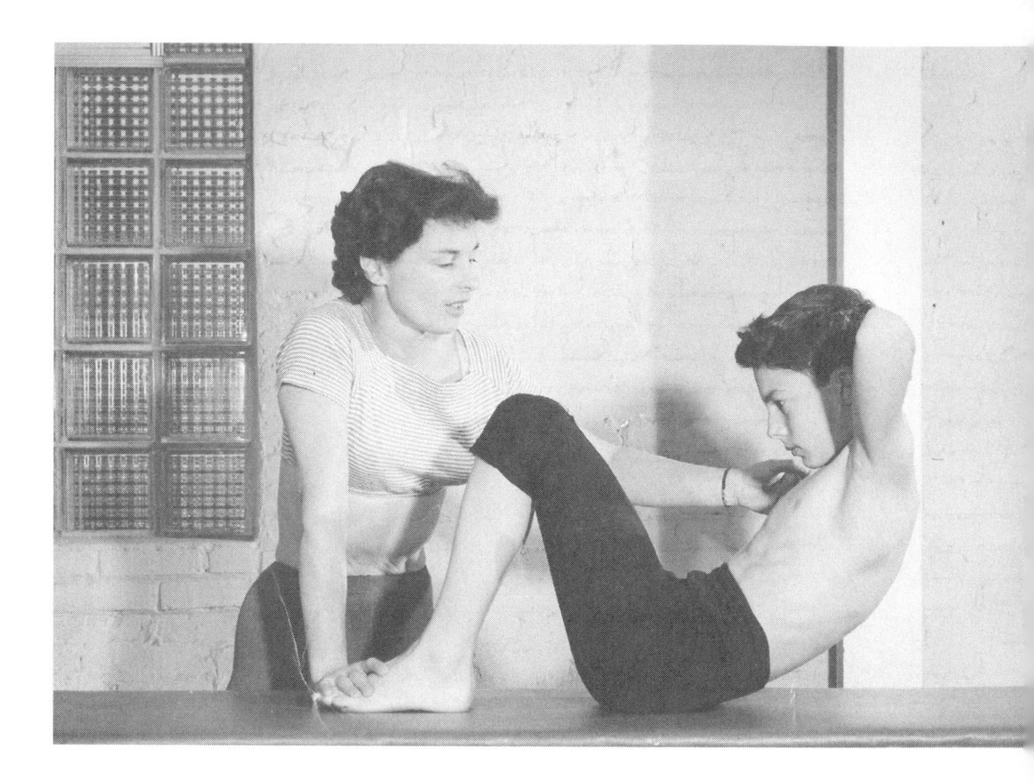

11. Bonnie Prudden, renowned first as a rock climber, tested thousands of youth during the Cold War face-off with the Soviet Union. The alarming results, presented to Eisenhower, became known as "the report that shocked the president" and prompted the first Council of Fitness. Courtesy of Bonnie Prudden Myotherapy, Inc.

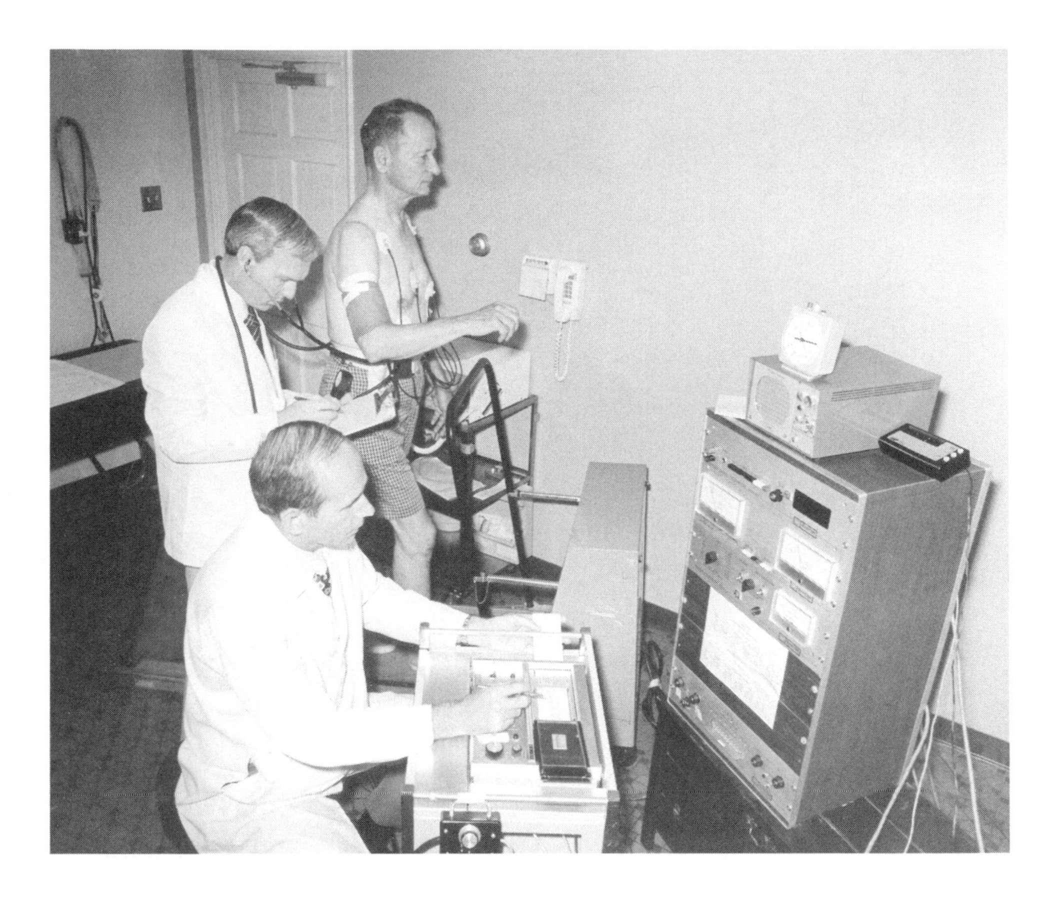

12. Dr. Kenneth Cooper (*foreground*) got America up and moving with his 1968 best seller, *Aerobics*. Naysayers warned his early treadmill test, the key to measuring cardiovascular activity, could kill the people he tested. Courtesy of Cooper Aerobics.

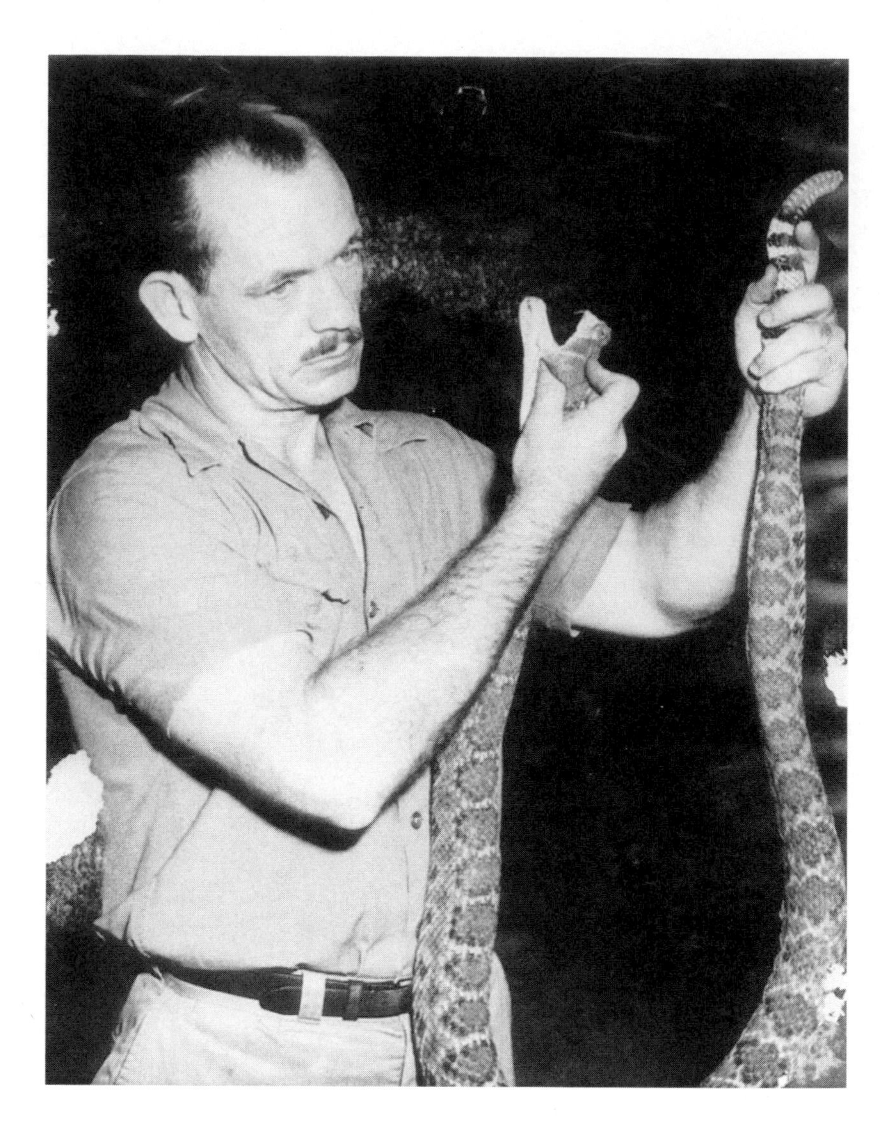

13. Arthur Jones, the inventor of the Nautilus machine, during his days as a big-game hunter and host of television's *Wild Cargo*. Pugnacious and brilliant, he summed up his favorite pursuits: "Younger women, faster airplanes, and bigger crocodiles." Courtesy of Gary Jones.

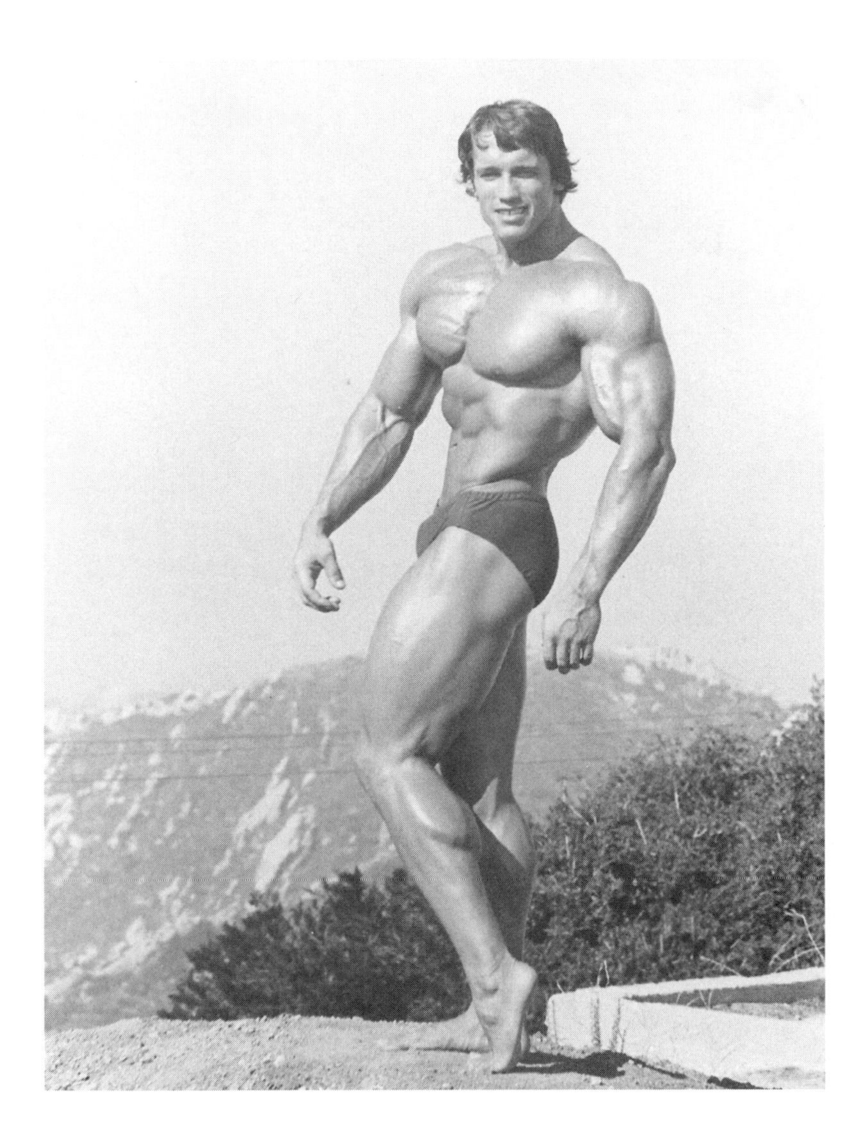

14. Naked women posed on his shoulders, and competitors quaked: Arnold Schwarzenegger, the "Austrian Oak," in his prime on "Muscle Rock, California." Courtesy of the Stark Center/University of Texas. Photograph by John Balik.

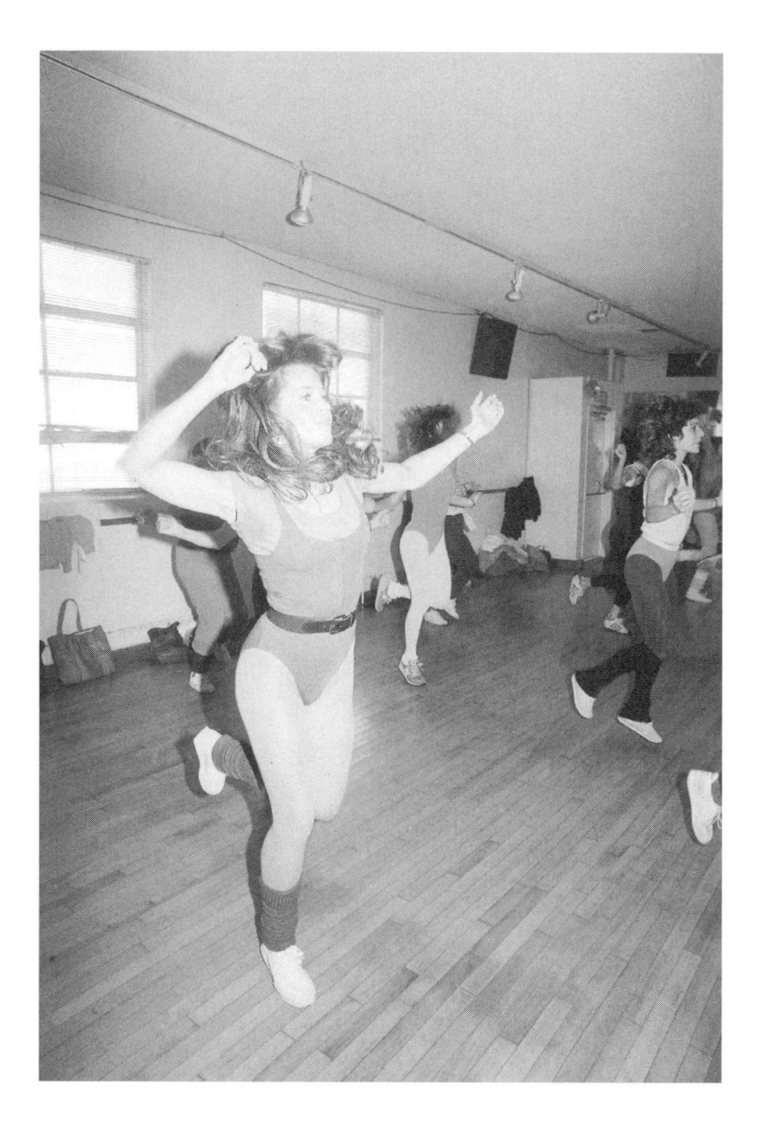

15. Jane Fonda used her star power to start a revolution in group exercise. Her first *Workout* book sold two million copies in hardcover: her videos launched the VCR industry. Courtesy of AP. Photo by Reed Saxon.

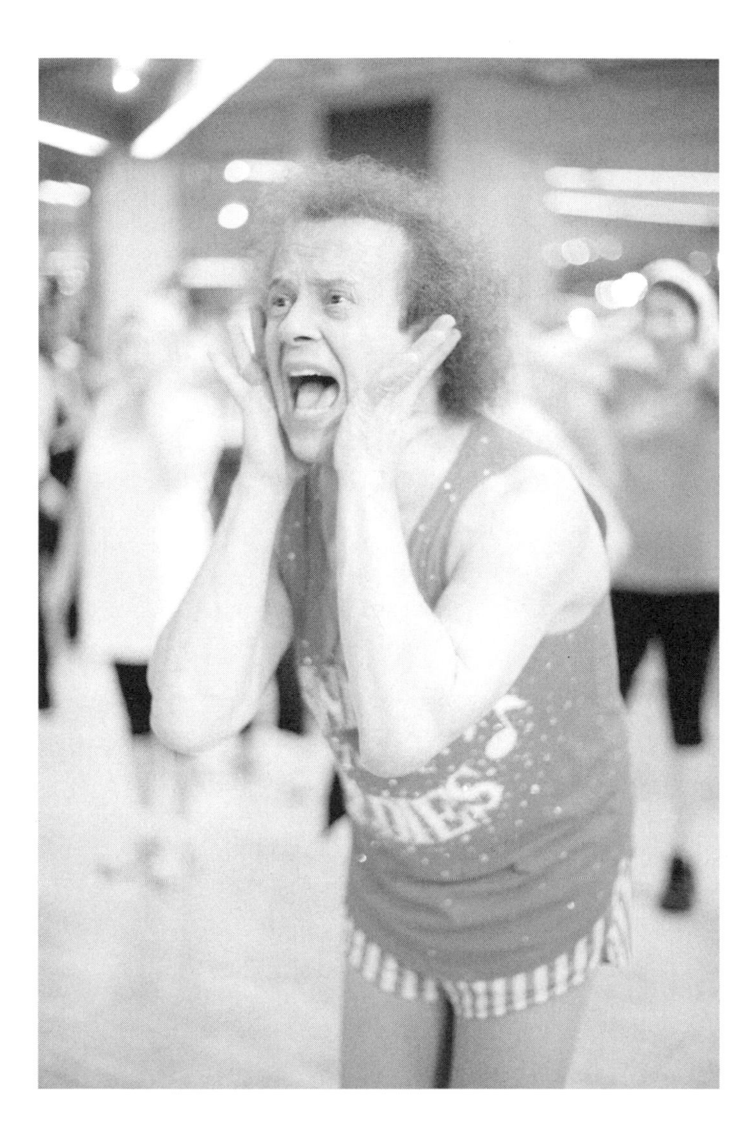

16. The former New Orleans fattie Richard Simmons reveled in his role as camp clown. The longest-running act in fitness, he convinced millions of out-of-shape women to shed inhibitions and get serious about their health. © Stephanie Diani/CORBIS.

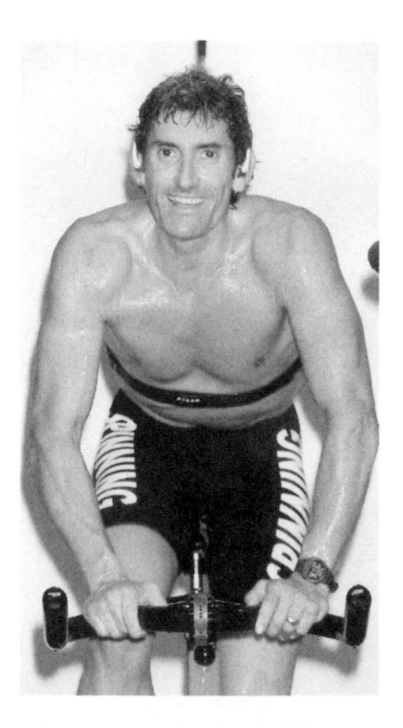

17. Johnny Goldberg, a.k.a. "Johnny G.," transformed group exercise when he unleashed Spinning on health clubs. The promo brochure called the forty-minute class "part Tour de France, part yoga, and part 12th century torture chamber." Courtesy of Johnny Goldberg.

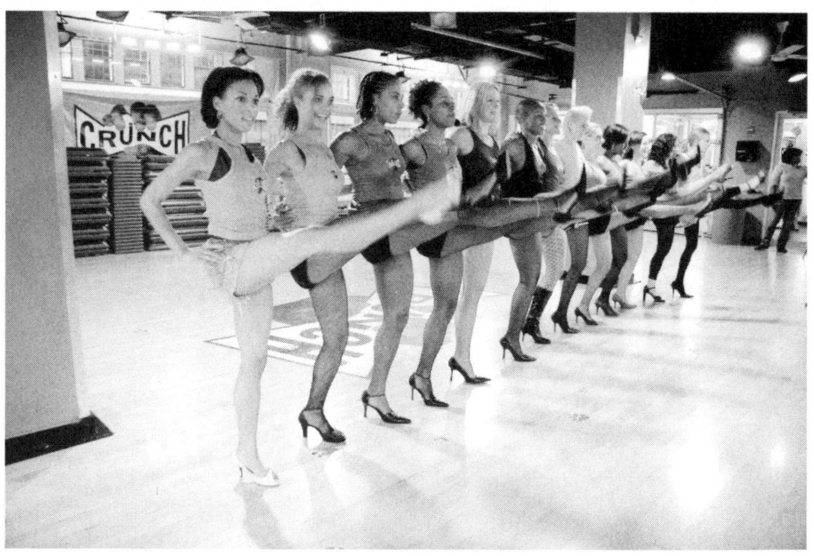

18. As the century drew to a close, the pursuit of fitness increasingly focused on clubs, where social bonding in the studio was a prime draw. Crunch Fitness pioneered the way with its "no judgments" brand and fun, sexy workouts such as "Stiletto Strength." Courtesy of Crunch Fitness.

was more a fringe irritant to Hoffman at its inception. In part it was overshadowed by a host of other organizations that soon sprang up, many in response to the first Mr. Universe contest held in 1947 in Philadelphia, then the following year in London. In no particular order, these tongue-twisters included the International Weightlifting Federation — also known as the Federation Internationale Halterophile, due to its French roots — the British Amateur Weightlifters Association, and the National Amateur Bodybuilders Association. Names changed; alliances were struck; backroom politics argued. The ultimate triumph of the IFBB owed much to the growing acceptance — or adulation — of the purely muscular body and its embrace by celebrities and mainstream media. To escape the confusion of titles, Weider resolved to create his own contest and gave full credit to his wife, Betty, for pushing the idea, if not the name "Mr. Olympia." That was owed to a rare night of drinking with Betty and a bodybuilder, Larry Scott. "While Betty and Larry kicked around names, none of which I liked, I looked at the bottle of beer in front of me — Olympics beer, from Olympia, Washington. That was my 'Eureka!' moment. I think maybe the gods intervened to put the perfect majestic word for the new contest in front of me."

The first Mr. Olympia contest was held at the Brooklyn Academy of Music in September 1965, the tail end of a program that featured the Miss Americana beauty pageant, the IFBB's Mr. America, and Mr. Universe. It drew only three contestants but soon took off, attracting bigger crowds and bigger names. Weider, meanwhile, was flexing his entrepreneurial muscle. He added more magazine titles. He began selling equipment. He promoted his training methods. The good times lacked only one thing, as he would write in *Brothers of Iron*: "Now that the IFBB had a worldwide reach and Mr. Olympia was up and running, bodybuilding was ready for its own superstar."

That person came to Weider's attention the day his London agent urged him to take a look at this "great big youngster from Austria" who had just won the London Mr. Universe contest. He had been featured in a story by John Grimek in Hoffman's *Muscular Development*, following a picture of him on the previous month's cover, but that was it. He had never been to the United States. His ties and possible allegiance to York and archrival Hoffman evidently stoked Weider's interest, and he invited the Austrian to appear at the IFBB Mr. Olympia contest in New York City.

In the July 1968 issue of *Muscle Builder/Power*, he put the man on the cover, along with a profile. In the same issue Ben Weider further hyped the upcoming contest with a fake description of the giant's arrival: "He's wearing dark glasses and an immense overcoat to cloak his enormous body. But the disguise does little good as his flaming blond hair gives him away. He's halfway up the steps when someone screamed, 'That's Arnold Schwarzenegger!'"

Ultimately, Schwarzenegger passed up the Mr. Olympia contest in favor of a less competitive Mr. Universe competition scheduled right after the New York event. It was there, in Miami Beach, that Joe Weider got his firsthand look at the man and professed to be "not so overwhelmed." "What he had in size," Weider noted, "he lacked in definition and overall proportion . . . heavy and smooth . . . underdeveloped in the legs, no abs, no delts, and white as a ghost. . . . To be blunt, I thought Arnold was overrated."

He soon changed his mind. Arnold had potential, he decided after watching him stare with rapt fixation at the contest's IFBB trophy. This was a man with resolve and the indomitable will to win. It would lead Weider to declaim: "When the student is ready, the teacher appears. When Arnold Schwarzenegger was ready, Joe Weider appeared. And when bodybuilding was ready, Arnold appeared. The moment was right because I made it right."

ARNOLD TO THE RESCUE

In Weider's world, and in a segment of the fitness culture, bodybuilding remained an iconic pursuit for men who equated masculinity with muscles. For others, the practice of working out with iron to develop a bulging chest and mighty arms had lost its cachet. Even Jack LaLanne, the push-up king, promoted a livelier all-round workout on television. Scrawny youth still sent in money for booklets on Dynamic Tension, but Charles Atlas had long since retreated to Florida and a solitary life of beach runs. He was scarcely missed. For many, the practice of turning one's body into a so-called work of art had increasingly been viewed with some suspicion, if not outright scorn. In 1974 the writer Charles Gaines attempted to rectify the sport's questionable image with his lively coffee-table book, *Pumping Iron*, which featured striking pictures by photographer George Butler, but Gaines was the first to acknowledge that the glory days were fast slipping away. "Bodybuilding has advertised itself with consummate tackiness," he wrote in the book's introduction, "confining itself to the back pages of pulp magazines and, in the national consciousness, to the same shadowy corners occupied by dildos and raincoat exhibitionists. . . . The composite picture that seems to have emerged from them, of bodybuilders as narcissistic, coordinatively [*sic*] helpless muscle-heads with suspect sexual preferences, has done little to promote the sport."

The "suspect sexual preference" of bodybuilders had long been a commonplace view, though, in truth, there was never much evidence that musclemen were any more homosexual than the rest of the population. The charge rested more on their presumed appeal to gays, which seemed undeniable, if less than conclusive. As far back as Sandow, women, too, had found men's outsized muscles an object of erotic fascination. Gaines, an apologist for hetero sex, described a girl accidentally backing into a major muscleman at a bar one night in the early seventies: "He caught her. She turned to him, her head just above the level of his waist, and began to feel him experimentally. She felt, paused, felt a little higher. 'Je-sus Christ,' she shrieked at her friends. 'Come *feel* this. Look at this goddam body!'"

The sexual appeal of bodybuilders (for those who found them appealing) was no big mystery. There was the physical allure: the visual treat of developed muscles. There was the appeal of what this conveyed: strength, the core masculine ideal, the suggestion of power and dominance. Finally, there was the erotic promise: these were men who were obviously consumed with the physical and, most particularly, with their own bodies. They shaved them, oiled them, regarded them with admiration in mirrors, posed in the skimpiest possible briefs. Whether this obsessive self-regard made for a healthy attitude toward sexual relations or resulted in actual performance was a matter of conjecture. Whether it supported a clinical case of narcissism depended on how one defined narcissism.

Christopher Lasch, in his epochal study of the subject, *The Culture of Narcissism*, took pains to detail its true nature. The narcissist suffered not from rampant self-love but from the inability to develop a separate sense of others. Narcissus was drowned not because he was so enamored of his image but because he mistook the watery reflection for himself.

Bodybuilders, in fact, were well aware of "other" selves — at least as regarding their tight-knit, bonded community. No sport demanded such a Herculean solo effort, and musclemen as a group tended to be loyal and generous in their appreciation of each other's work and sacrifice.

Outsiders had less invested. Not a few psychologists questioned the presumed satisfaction behind the big smiles and cheerful virility of the musclemen. Of course, they had much to be grateful for. Many had used the sport to overcome a childhood blighted by illness, weight problems, and injury. Others — a much broader population — found it a means to combat insults, bullying, and insecurity. But were they in fact happy? Had building a better body erased feelings of unworthiness? Several studies would find that bodybuilders, despite the trappings of confidence, continued to suffer from low self-esteem. A professor at Vanderbilt, Bianca Hitt, called it "Reverse Anorexia." Women — the vast majority of anorexics — tried to overcome a poor self-image by starving themselves to more closely resemble the unrealistic models in popular magazines. Bodybuilders did the opposite. They piled on muscle mass, and they obsessively manipulated what went into their body — all in the interests of control that eluded them in the rest of their lives. At root the insecurities lingered — and so did a sense of isolation. "Bodybuilding attracts loners because of the high degree of individualism in the sport. The competitive bodybuilder," wrote Hitt, "like the individual with anorexia nervosa, engages in a social comparison process which may cause him or her to avoid others out of a sense of inadequacy."

As the seventies arrived, the habit of creating huge blocks of carved muscle seemed more susceptible than ever to charges that it was a superficial and solipsistic pursuit. The Hoffman-Weider battles had tilted in favor of Weider; bodybuilding, the showy art of posing and merely looking magnificent, was triumphing over the ugly functional grunt work of weight lifting, a sport now dominated by the Eastern-bloc countries and their state-supported champions. Weider himself had moved his company headquarters from its proletarian backwater in New Jersey to the sun-drenched capital of hedonism, Los Angeles. This was the dawn of the Me Decade, as it would become labeled by Tom Wolfe, an era of self-absorption when the mirrored glass of gyms seemed to reflect a love of self and not much more. "The '70s was the decade in which people put emphasis on the skin, on the surface, rather on the root of things,"

Norman Mailer complained in 1979. "It was the decade in which image became preeminent because nothing deeper was going on."

But all of this was about to change (at least the demeaning of muscle), thanks entirely to one man. In the space of a few years, Arnold Schwarzenegger would single-handedly rescue bodybuilding from marginalization. He would give it a flash of celebrity glamour it had never enjoyed in its heyday. And he would stake his claim on a beach that would soon become the most famous playground in fitness.

Muscle Beach in Santa Monica, the old playground, had rolled up its last mats in the late 1950s. Though so instrumental in showcasing an earlier generation of muscleman, its time had come and gone. Gymnastics and acrobatics, such fun to watch on the sand, seemed the sport of an earlier, more innocent era. Live entertainment, in general, had given up ground to television as a mass-entertainment medium, and the eye-popping pyramids of bodies seemed less gripping than quaint. The musclemen, however, had not entirely vanished, and the new practitioners simply migrated south — to Venice Beach.

Venice was not, at least at first, the carefree playground of Santa Monica. It was a down-at-the-heels, seedy conglomeration of tourist stands and beach bums. The locus of activity was a small enclosed area called "the Pit" or "the Pen," a small fenced-in area with barbells and dumbbells. For its hard-core cadre of bodybuilders, the indoor training took place in the no-nonsense gym on nearby Venice Avenue that would become world famous as "the mecca of bodybuilding" or, more simply, as Gold's Gym.

The man behind Gold's, Joe Gold, was a working-class stiff with few pretensions of glamour. Born in 1928, the son of a Jewish junk man, he grew up in the tough working-class slums of East Los Angeles. His family rented summer vacation bungalows near Muscle Beach, and he became a regular at the Weight Pen, playing beach volleyball and lifting weights. Following a stint in the Philippines during World War II, where he was wounded in a torpedo strike, he joined the Merchant Marines, sailing around the world and always with a set of weights. He became a competitive bodybuilder in the 1950s and an occasional movie stuntman, and he joined Mae West's nightclub troupe with his musclemen pals. Gyms were scarce then — Los Angeles had only three clubs — and dingy at best; at the famed Dungeon, even power lifters left their wallets at home. "The guys had nowhere to go when Muscle Beach closed," he explained, "and they needed a place to work out. That's how Gold's Gym got its start."

Gold opened his gym in 1965. A skilled machinist, he welded most of the equipment himself from scrap metal and designed unique machines that would appeal to serious strongmen, calling his gym "the first made specifically for bodybuilders." He had little interest in attracting anyone else. He never bought ads in the LA papers and refused to list it in the Yellow Pages. There was no sign on the narrow street facade, the gym's windows were sealed, and Gold usually kept the front door locked. Inside, the gym ran back one hundred feet, with a narrow staircase that led to a small loft with a changing area and shower. The view was daunting. "If you got up on the second-floor balcony and looked down, you'd think you were looking at hell, at Dante's Inferno," recalled bodybuilding journalist Dick Tyler. "The steam literally coming off the floor from the sweat and yelling and clanking plates. All of these guys training and the screaming. 'One more set!' 'One more set, you faggot!'"

Gold was no businessman, he had no interest in growing the brand, and in 1970 he sold the gym and the right to his name and went back to sea as a commercial sailor. He thus failed to reap the publicity bonanza that would soon attach to his gym—as the site of a documentary that starred the almighty Austrian who started training at Gold's shortly after his arrival in California in 1968.

It would be impossible to overestimate the influence Arnold Schwarzenegger had on the world of bodybuilding and fitness in general. His subsequent success, as a film star and politician, owed much to his willful ambition and a personality that was equal parts charm and cunning. But all began with the body, a body that was so massive and magnificently developed it brought gasps from fans and quaking cases of nerves from competitors. Not for nothing was he known as the "Austrian Oak."

He was born in the Austrian village of Thal, the son of the local police chief, Gustav, whose intimidating size and dominant manner made for a tense childhood. In addition to beatings—"My hair was pulled. I was hit with belts. So was the kid next door. It was just the way it was"—he had to contend with an older brother, Meinhard, enthroned as his father's favorite. He rebelled at any opportunity and found what nurture he could from his emotionally supportive mother. Like tens of thousands,

Gustav joined the Nazi Party, though not all took that allegiance a step further, as Gustav did by volunteering to join the storm troopers, four months after the Reich's annexation of Austria. When Gustav died, Schwarzenegger failed to attend his father's funeral, either because of long-standing bitterness (one version) or because he was in the midst of training for a bodybuilding contest (his own version, as it appeared in *Pumping Iron*). Nor did he attend the funeral of his brother, Meinhard, who died drunk in a car accident in 1971 after a short, dissolute life as a playboy and habitual con man.

A multisport athlete, he picked up his first barbell at the age of thirteen when his soccer coach took him to a local gym; he soon dropped all other sports to devote himself to bodybuilding. His idols, whom he saw in magazines and onscreen at the local movie theater, were Reg Park, Steve Reeves, and Johnny Weissmuller. Determined to become the greatest bodybuilder in the world, he won two successive Mr. Universe titles, in 1967 and 1968, first amateur and then professional, and set his eyes on the ultimate crown in bodybuilding, the Mr. Olympia contest, sponsored by Weider's IFBB. To win, however, would require wresting the title from the formidable world champion, Sergio Oliva. Wary of an immediate showdown, he chose to compete in the 1968 Mr. Universe contest in Miami.

Weider's version of Schwarzenegger's first trip to the States, not surprisingly, tends to emphasize his own proactive role. Other facts suggest that Schwarzenegger played a part in plotting this major step by agreeing to appear in *Strength and Health*, the magazine of Weider's nemesis, York patriarch Bob Hoffman, figuring an alliance with Hoffman would land him the bigger fish, Weider. And so it did, according to Frank Colombu, Schwarzenegger's longtime bodybuilding pal: "[Arnold] told Joe, 'Hoffman wants me to go to York,' and Joe went crazy."

Schwarzenegger's debut in America did not go as planned. He not only placed second to Frank Zane, who was three inches shorter and sixty-five pounds lighter, but had to suffer the contest's emcee announcing the recently crowned and repeat winner of Mr. Olympia: "The one and only unchallenged king of bodybuilding—Sergio Oliva." Shaken and briefly humbled, he accepted Weider's offer to come to California, where Weider promised to set him up in an apartment, pay for gym sessions, and promote Arnold in his magazines.

Both men had much to gain from the arrangement, a fact that never escaped Schwarzenegger. "He had contacted me because I could be useful to him," he wrote in his 1977 autobiography, *Arnold: The Education of a Body Builder.* "I accepted that. But I knew he could be useful to me. There were still a number of important goals before me, and this man could help me realize them."

The partnership sent both their careers into orbit. Weider finally had his star, whom he trained and promoted relentlessly in his magazines. Schwarzenegger had his benefactor, who, as promised, supplied an apartment, a modest weekly salary, and a membership at Gold's Gym. At Schwarzenegger's urging, Weider also brought over Arnold's pal, Columbu, and the two friends moved into a larger apartment that quickly became a hub for bodybuilders, as well as a source of income. When the two men asked Weider for extra money, the publisher told them to write articles for his magazine. Instead, they bought a tape recorder and debriefed their muscled pals while the men ate grilled steaks and drank red wine on the patio. Then they took the tapes to negotiate with Weider. "Here, Joe, give us the money, fifteen hundred dollars," Arnold said. "Fifteen hundred dollars?" Weider replied incredulously. "Fifteen hundred? You guys just made the tapes. No, maybe a thousand."

As crafty as Weider, the men switched to shorter tapes, turning one into five, a scheme that worked fine until Weider finally lost patience. "You know, I give you guys an opportunity to become champions and big stars," Weider sputtered. "I put you on the cover. And then I get these tapes and they're short and the tapes don't talk about training, they talk about how much you guys are drinking."

The two left empty-handed. Like other dealings with Weider, however, it left the ever-opportunistic Schwarzenegger with another lesson on making it big in America. As he would later muse: "I found out right away that Joe had two personalities. The warm, beautiful human Joe Weider in his private life, and the shrewd businessman at the office. I admire both sides of the man. Business fascinates me. I get caught up in the whole idea that it's a game to make money and to make money make more money. Joe Weider is a wizard at it, and I liked being able to watch him operate."

Schwarzenegger was a fast operator himself. Though he spoke only fractured English on his arrival, he quickly enrolled in evening classes at a community college and at UCLA. He launched a bricklaying business with Columbu, much in demand after the 1971 earthquake, then used the profits to start a mail-order company. He bought real estate. He became a phenomenon at Gold's Gym, where Gaines, watching in awe as the man did his sets and routines, called him "the best bodybuilder alive, and very possibly the most perfectly developed man in the history of the world."

Gold's had been an intense place before, but Arnold upped the ante. "Nine-thirty, sharp, he'd walk through that door, and everyone threw more plates on the bar," remembers Eddie Guiliani, the 1974 Mr. America (short division) and an early Gold's workhorse. "He'd ride you all day and the day after, too. Arnold saw everything, and he didn't forget." You had to impress him, no matter the cost. "[There were] guys fainting after squats, guys throwing up in the alley, he was at a whole other level."

The gym was the locus of other activity. Most of the serious bodybuilders dosed themselves with the first crude anabolic steroid drugs—Dianabol tables and Deca-Durabolin shots, a combo that grew muscles but also compromised heart walls. The results were plain to see in Weider's magazines, now including *Flex*, where the 1970s iron men soon dwarfed their earlier counterparts. Gold's was also the hub for a lively traffic in male models and the occasional recruitment for Colt Studios, the producer of pornographic films, straight and gay. The gym was rife with hustlers. "Not everyone did it, but the list of guys who did would cover every title," said Ken Sprague, the new owner of Gold's. "Up to and including Mr. Olympia."

Outside Gold's Arnold and his pals created a public sensation on the sands of Muscle Beach in Venice, which, unlike its earlier incarnation in Santa Monica, was home to more overt displays of sexuality. This was the seventies, and objectification, though spurned by the rising tide of feminists, was part and parcel of the new openness. A fit body invited inspection—and more. Women in bikinis and halter tops openly eyed the muscleman or sidled up close for a feel or personal business. Arnold lapped up the attention, cheerfully posing with bare-breasted women perched on his shoulders; nor did he claim to be bothered by the evident interest of men. "When a homosexual looks at a bodybuilder, I don't have any problem against that," he declared. "I would probably stare the same way if Raquel Welch or Brigitte Bardot walked by. If I see a girl with big tits, I'm going to stare and stare. And I'm going to think in my mind what I'm going to do with her if I would have her. The same is true of the homosexual."

Schwarzenegger dominated the world of competitive bodybuilding in the early seventies. In addition to his massive body and finely cut muscles, he became a master at the art of posing. He studied how opponents ran their routine; he exploited their flaws; he undercut their confidence with sly digs. Onstage he would explode as he hit his poses, stunning the audience and overwhelming the competition. He finally conquered his nemesis, Sergio Oliva, winning the 1972 Mr. Olympia title in Essen, Germany. He then won the next five consecutive Mr. Olympia titles, an extraordinary record. His name, however, was about to get bigger—much bigger.

His physique and wit had already landed him on television with Merv Griffin and even Lucille Ball. In 1974 he joined Gaines and Butler on *The Today Show* with Barbara Walters to promote their upcoming book, *Pumping Iron*, which went through four printings before its 1974 on-sale date. Never one to balk at self-promotion, he even agreed to be photographed nude for *Cosmopolitan* by Francesco Scavullo, joining Burt Reynolds as the magazine's only male centerfolds. He made his Hollywood debut in the film *Stay Hungry*. Based on Gaines's novel of that name, starring Sally Fields and Jeff Bridges and directed by Bob Rafelson, it was an eccentric mix of comedy and drama set in the "New South." Arnold looked altogether comfortable as the resident bodybuilder at an offbeat gym, romancing a quirky Fields and showing off his posing chops at an IFBB Mr. Universe contest. The most memorable scene was the wave of near-naked bodybuilders who ran through the town streets, dodging traffic and jumping on car roofs, but the film was only a modest success and quickly vanished.

Not Arnold. He had planned to retire from professional bodybuilding after his fifth Mr. Olympia title but was persuaded to go for one more by Gaines, who needed a real-life event to cap his planned documentary of *Pumping Iron*. When Gaines ran out of money to complete the edit, he concocted an artsy fund-raising "seminar" at the Whitney Museum of Art in Manhattan, which the museum called "The Articulate Muscle: The Male Body in Art" and featured Arnold and two bodybuilding pals on raised rotating discs.

Gaines and photographer Butler had anticipated several hundred people. Instead, five thousand showed up, so mobbing the ticket tables that money was tossed on the floor in piles. The crowd was a mix of sober fine-arts types, thrilled voyeurs, and media headliners, among them Candice Bergen, on assignment for *The Today Show*. The evening produced enough cash to finish the edit—and Bergen provided the perfect anecdote. Riding in a postevent limousine with Butler, she remarked that the oiled Austrian had just exhausted his fifteen minutes of fame. Butler disagreed and predicted, "Arnold Schwarzenegger is going to be Governor of California"—to which Bergen laughed and retorted, "Sure . . . and Ronald Reagan is going to be President of the United States!"

What few predicted was the success of Gaines's film, *Pumping Iron*. With all the training footage shot at Gold's Gym, it produced a fascinating window into a cult sport, showcasing muscles, sex, and ambition. The top-billed drama, of course, was the great Arnold going for one last win against the upstart giant, Lou Ferrigno, a sympathetic but doomed combatant. A lone, inarticulate East Coaster who trained in a dingy Brooklyn gym, hectored by his domineering real-life dad (largely put up to the role by Gaines), Ferrigno was no match for Arnold—certainly not in the hilarious dressing-room banter that destroyed his confidence. When Arnold mounted the winner's platform at Durbin, South Africa, he had secured not only another line in the record books but his future as the slyest of macho male stars. Never again would all bodybuilders be dismissed as dumb hormonal freaks. Ferrigno would eventually take some solace from his Hollywood turn as the Incredible Hulk. As he noted in *Pumping Iron*'s twenty-fifth-anniversary "added footage" bonus on the DVD, Durbin opened his eyes to the fun he could be having living like Arnold. On the same DVD, other Gold's alumni reminisced about the great times in the seventies and the friends they still talked to. "As for Arnold Schwarzenegger," the narrator drily concluded, "he went on to make a few bucks in the movie business."

STAR POWER

Arnold was not the first male actor to exploit a bared physique. The pulp stars of the fifties and sixties had gained a measure of fame by stripping off their shirts. Victor Mature and Robert Mitchum often flaunted their chests. Burt Lancaster's bathing-suit beach scene with Deborah Kerr in *From Here to Eternity* came close to scandal status in the buttoned-up fifties. But none of them, not even Lancaster—a former circus acrobat—had the cut muscles that now seemed so sexy. It was left to Sylvester Stallone, the "Italian Stallion," to bring that look to the big screen. The warrior workouts in *Rocky* had audiences cheering for the all-American fighter and left a few other actors taking nervous glances in their dressing-room mirror.

Notable among them was John Travolta, who was slated to star in the much-hyped sequel to *Saturday Night Fever*. Only now, instead of a laid-back disco guy, he was cast as a dance instructor. Worse, the movie, *Staying Alive*, was being directed by, of all people, Stallone. Travolta could sing, he could act, he could definitely dance—but he was not in Rocky shape, not even close. Months before shooting was scheduled to begin, he was in Aspen, Colorado, starring in a summer-stock play, when he met an athletic consultant at the nearby Snowmass Club. "I couldn't have been a better pilot project," said Travolta.

The Travolta "project" fell to Dan Isaacson, a short and fit midwesterner who managed one of the country's first multisports clubs in Denver. Like Travolta, Isaacson flew planes, and the two men hit it off. For three months he trained Travolta—supervising daily workouts, monitoring what he ate, taking off fat, and adding muscle. When Travolta showed up on the *Staying Alive* set, he was a man transformed; even Stallone was impressed. Travolta was so pleased he persuaded Isaacson to move to Los Angeles, where he put up money for a twelve-hundred-square-foot studio that Isaacson packed with fifty thousand dollars' worth of equipment. Before you could say "personal trainer," Travolta's movie star pals and Hollywood bigwigs were clamoring for time.

Mickey Rourke needed to look buff as the sexy stud in *9½ Weeks*. Linda Evans wanted to perk up her sex appeal in *Dynasty*. David Hasselhoff, star of *Knight Rider*, got his number, and so did David Geffen, who recruited Larry Gelbart and Irwin Winkler. Isaacson met Burt Reynolds at a party. Christopher Reeve had to trim the beef he had packed on for *Superman*—and flew Isaacson to Williamstown, Massachusetts, where he was playing summer stock; weeks of punishing hands-on training, and Reeve was a convert. He worked with comedians—Billy Crystal, Robin Williams, Martin Short. Danny Sullivan, the glamorous race-car driver, hired Isaacson to help restore his battered body after a near-fatal wreck in his Porsche.

Isaacson ministered to them all, sculpting their bodies and gingerly coddling their egos. "If Mickey Rourke requests an after-midnight workout, Isaacson opens the gym," wrote a reporter for *Time*. "If Danny Sullivan asks him to fly to Indianapolis, he gets on a jet. If Travolta likes new sweats and shoes for every workout, Isaacson supplies them."

Some he trained at home, some at his Malibu gym. Travolta suggested he move his equipment into a room on the lot at Fox, the studio producing *Staying Alive*. "I asked him, 'You sure that's okay?' He said, 'Sure, just don't make a big deal of it.'" He trained twenty clients a day, including Marilu Henner, Jon Voigt, Olivia Newton-John, running from 6:00 a.m. workouts in Malibu to Fox—until the day he showed up and found the door padlocked. Apparently, no one had cleared the studio gym with Fox boss Joe Wizan. When the snafu got cleared up, Isaacson focused on "bringing fitness to the studio lot—that was my goal." He achieved it in 1986 when Paramount became the first studio to build a personal-training center—"the cornerstone of corporate facilities in America," said Isaacson, and he was likely right.

Isaacson, despite his glamorous clientele, kept his work grounded in fitness basics; his book *The Equation* was an informed and detailed guide to eating right and measuring body fat. He never exploited his star connections and made only one workout video—as the male counterpart to Jane Fonda. Pictured on the box's cover, he was the only man to ever costar with Fonda. He might have made more of a splash had not another trainer emerged in the celebrity ether first.

His name was Jake Steinfeld, and, like Isaacson, who got his start with Travolta, his fame stemmed from a chance meeting with another of filmdom's iconic names. However, unlike Isaacson, who was relatively modest in demeanor, Steinfeld was a barrel-chested dynamo of self-promotion, as funny as he was fit, a Borscht Belt comedian with the body and propulsion of an NFL linebacker.

He hailed from Baldwin, Long Island, and had landed in Los Angeles with hopes of becoming Mr. America. "A fat kid with a stutter" is how he characterized his early years until he discovered weight training, his life's passion. Three months into his freshman year at an upstate New York college, he had his "aha" moment on a frigid lacrosse field. "It was hailing, starting to snow, and I thought, 'What am I *doing*?' I went back to my dorm and called home and said, 'Mom, I'm going to go to California and become a bodybuilder.' Silence. Then: 'Herbie, pick up the phone and talk to your kid. I'm putting my head in the oven.'"

With his parents' wary blessing, he went to pursue his dream in Los Angeles. It did not last long. Competing in the 1978 Mr. Southern California contest, he placed second to "a guy that was on steroids. It was a time when dinosaurs roamed the earth, when big men were still the flavor, but I wasn't into taking drugs. I loved working out, I wanted to get huge, but I saw what the world was like."

He became a club bouncer; he landed a gig as the Incredible Hulk for Universal Studio tours. He met an actress, the wife of Keith Carradine, who was about to shoot a Club Med commercial and needed to get in bikini shape. She was frightened of weights, so he improvised with a towel pull and broomstick. Thrilled with the results, she told a friend, who wanted to give her boyfriend a special birthday gift. A few days later he showed up with his towel and broomstick at a Beverly Hills mansion, and Steven Spielberg answered the door.

One thing led to another—"I became famous by association," he would later admit—and soon Steinfeld had his own stable of stars, a roster that included Harrison Ford and Barbra Streisand and Margot Kidder and Priscilla Presley. He traveled on the Warners company jet "with the great Steve Ross." He trained Michael Jackson and Bette Midler. "It happened so fast. People started saying, 'My God, you look great, what are you doing?' They'd say 'This guy Jake comes to my house with a broomstick and a towel and a chair, tells some funny stories.' They'd say, 'Sounds great, what's his phone?' I'd never listed a phone, which gave me even more of a mystique, so people said, 'Who *is* this guy? *Get* him!'"

He made up T-shirts for select clients. The back read "The Steinfeld Method." Spielberg told him, "'The Steinfeld Method'? What are you, a gynecologist? Get rid of it. You're a lifestyle, a brand.' So I changed it to 'Body by Jake.' If my name were Murray, it would have been 'Body by Murray.'"

He trademarked "Trainer to the Stars" along with his motto, "Don't Quit!," and began doing thirty-second "Fitness Breaks" for the new cable sports channel ESPN with Hollywood starlets and more home props. "I'd go, 'Here's your fitness tip, today, bicep curls. You need two cans of Mama's Tomato Paste. Meet Brenda, Miss April, and here's Miss June.'

Beautiful blue sky, a few motivational moments, then, 'Remember, don't quit! Have a great day.' And out."

He starred in his own syndicated sitcom on the Family Channel, *Big Brother Jake*, which ran four years. He had bit parts in movies. He published a book (*Body by Jake*), put out a record and video (*Body by Jake*), and did promotional TV spots (*Body by Jake*). "The only problem," he explained at the time, "is: How do I keep up the whole Body by Jake mystique—you know, the celebrity clients, the unlisted number?"

Then that unlisted phone rang one morning, and a man on the other end said, "I just read about you in *People*. I want to start a 24-hour fitness network. My name is Ted Turner."

Steinfeld signed up and became a cable personality on CNN. He left shortly before Turner met the actress who had made America "feel the burn"—and launched a business that would bring Body by Jake into untold millions of households. Personal training had made him brand famous; the infomercial would make him rich.

WOMEN ARE STRONG, TOO

The province of looking buff and strong was dominated by men, and the reasons were more or less obvious. Physiologically, women were not endowed with the same muscle mass as men. Aesthetically, the feminine ideal, varied as it was, stressed grace over strength, beauty over brawn. Men who built up their bodies could be seen as enhancing—or, at worst, exaggerating—the male ideal; women who packed on muscle were distorting what God had decreed.

This view, not surprisingly, has been subjected to withering attacks from a small but vocal group of feminists, as well as enlightened members of both sexes. But history was not on their side, at least for a long time. In the nineteenth century women with muscles were largely confined to sideshow acts in circuses or vaudeville. Developed musculature was seen as "unsexing" a woman and likely—as described in an 1878 article in the *American Christian Review*—part of a nine-step path that led to sin and ruin. The so-called golden age of the early twentieth century featured the likes of Sandwina, who lifted three large men while on a bicycle, but did little to give strong women any mainstream recognition. When Macfadden staged a women's "physical culture contest" in conjunction with his men's headliner at Madison Square Garden, the women wore tight-fitting long underwear and were judged, wrote historian Jan Todd, "on general healthfulness and appearance rather than muscularity."

Not much changed in the next fifty years. Jack LaLanne allowed women to train at his 1936 Oakland gym and held an occasional "beauty contest" to encourage them. On Muscle Beach the women's contests bore such names as "Miss Body Beautiful" and "Miss Physical Fitness," and women were discouraged from poses that accentuated their muscles. Pudgy Stockton was virtually alone in attracting widespread publicity, and even Pudgy conformed to the male notion of shapeliness and a breezy, nonthreatening personality. As late as 1978 the disparaging of muscled women was evident when the bodybuilder and emcee Dennis Walters followed a straightforward report on a Mr. Universe main event with: "On to the fanny-swingers in the Miss World Physical Fitness Division."

In her book *Bodymakers* Leslie Heywood found much in the seventies that turned the tide and made such remarks sound archaic at best. Feminism, at least its "second wave," was gathering steam. Title IX brought women into sports; affirmative action helped bring equality to the workplace. Movie heroines — Sigourney Weaver in *Alien*, Farrah Fawcett in *Extremities* — created strong women role models. More statuesque models like Christie Brinkley and Cindy Crawford became popular. Heywood's 1998 book offered a dense if compelling look at the sociocultural forces that influenced the conflicted views of strong women, but Heywood — a professor of English as well as a bodybuilder — made only a single mention, and then just in passing, of the woman whom Todd crowns "the First Lady of Bodybuilding."

She was Doris Barrilleaux, born Doris Biering in Houston, Texas, in 1931. A mother of four by the time she was twenty-five, she began exercising when she could not hang from a playground's jungle-gym bars. She weight trained at a local gym, segregated from the men by a wooden partition, and had her revelatory moment when she sent a photo of herself to Bob Hoffman's *Strength and Health* — and was told the pose was "too masculine." A second submission, in which she is seated on a beach in a bikini, appeared in the February 1963 issue, accompanying a feature on "Family Fitness" run by the same editor who had rejected the first photo.

Barrilleaux was far from the highest-profile name in women's bodybuilding. That honor belonged to Lisa Lyon, a regular at Gold's Gym in Santa Monica, which hosted "the First Women's Bodybuilding Championships" at the Embassy Auditorium in 1978. To wild cheers Lyon walked off with the top prize. Bright, lithe, and attractive, a hit on TV talk shows, she cheerfully flaunted her muscles and more, posing for *Playboy* in 1980 and then for a 1983 Robert Mapplethorpe book of nude photographs called *Lady: Lisa Lyon*. Lyon, declared Heywood, was the first seriously sculpted woman to satisfy both men's desires and women's aspirations.

Barrilleaux was not the first to sponsor a women's bodybuilding contest. That credit goes to Henry McGhee, a bodybuilder and strength coach at the Canton, Ohio, YMCA, who promoted what is generally regarded as the first contest in which competitors were judged solely on muscularity: the June 17, 1978, "National Women's Physique Championship." But Barrilleaux was there that historic night. Forty-six years old, by then a Florida-based flight attendant and mother of six, she posed in a zebra-striped bikini and left the stage thrilled. "I sometimes wonder if I'd ever have had the gumption to begin running my own meets in Florida," she said, "if I hadn't entered Henry's meet."

The meets she ran, however, opened the door for women who wanted to build strength and pose on their own terms. Following McGhee's event, she connected with friends and formed the Superior Physique Association, the first bodybuilding organization to be run for women and by women. Within a year it was sponsoring almost a meet a month. She posed in contests. She lobbied for rules that would recognize a woman's unique muscularity. She served on "women's committees" at both the AAU and the IFBB and was tapped by Ben Weider to spearhead what became the American Federation of Women Bodybuilders (AFWB) under the IFBB umbrella. She bylined stories in Joe Weider's magazines and had a regular column, "Curves and Peaks," in Dan Lurie's *Muscle Training Illustrated*. She became adept at photography, and her pictures of bodybuilders appeared on close to two hundred magazine covers. In 1983 she published her second exercise book, *Forever Fit*.

The phenomenon of women's bodybuilding, meanwhile, fell victim to a tangle of controversy and politics, much of it relating to judging standards. The IFBB, which ran the Ms. Olympia contests, came under sharp criticism for its so-called femininity rules, among them a dictum to judges that competitors should not be "too big." A later decree in the 1990s announced the "20 percent rule," requiring that female athletes reduce their muscularity by 20 percent. As in the earliest days of visibly strong women, the images of highly developed female bodybuilders caused many to cringe, even as a new generation of enthusiasts had found a new source of sport and identity in lifting iron and becoming powerful. The best-known — six-time Ms. Olympia Cory Everson and the stunning Rachel McLish — were carved with impressive muscle while still maintaining a "feminine" look. The serious hobbyists, like Heywood, found their own efforts were the best reward. As Heywood wrote, "The gym is the world of gods and heroes, goddesses larger than life, a place of incantations where our bodies inflate and we shuffle off our out-of-gym bodies like discarded skins and walk about transformed."

But female bodybuilding, at least in its competitive ranks, would succumb to the same syndrome that came to dominate its male counterpart: the compulsion toward large. In part this was a result of the time put into training. Unlike men, who had been competing for decades, women were relatively new to the sport. "If you have an entirely new activity, it takes time for the body to adapt," said Todd. "When the [earliest] girls started to put on muscles, they still looked like gymnasts; they were fit and athletic." As years were added to training, however, the women came to resemble the men whose freakish physiques adorned the covers of muscle-head fan books like *Flex*. Everson, noted Todd, looked very different "before" than "after." Drugs and supplements likely added to an exaggerated musculature and led to a spooky gauntness and telltale tightened faces.

Though feminists were loath to criticize these women who, after all, were simply following the example of men who escaped censure for using testosterone, the result was the marginalization of female bodybuilding as a sport. Heywood, for one, came to disdain the new "steroid-based bodybuilding," which she tied to the "long-term detrimental health effects [that] can be read as a synecdoche for globalization and its 'grow-or-die' imperatives." Her epiphany came one night at a high school gym, where, backstage, she watched "women in black stilettos and red press-on nails, hair in big curlers," and was equally appalled by the leering men in the audience who came to gawk. "[It] was enough to make me turn away from female bodybuilding as a liberatory potential for women and girls, and instead turn to women's sports more generally." Recanting her early embrace of bodybuilding, she took up CrossFit, which she found "very addictive, very agro, and a great deal of fun."

Barrilleaux, the woman who had done so much to bring the sport into the mainstream, turned eighty in 2011—and continued to lift modest weights and ride her bicycle or swim daily.

CHAPTER 7

Pumping Up Business, 1980s–1990s

Clubs take over the landscape; Donahue Wildman takes over Tanny; the Age of Acronyms; the fun and power of groups; home alone

THE CLUB EXPLOSION

Looking around in the early twenty-first century, it is hard to imagine a time when the pursuit of fitness was separate from club membership. Health clubs today are ubiquitous. They range from owner-operated storefront studios to megaclubs that occupy acres and boast tennis courts, pools, and restaurants. The titleholder for "Most Amazing" is Red Lerelle's Health and Racquet Club in the unlikely town of Lafayette, Louisiana (population 113,656), a 185,000-square-foot megaplex with an outdoor water park and a membership base that includes more than 10 percent of the entire town. Elsewhere, they come in every imaginable stripe: city athletic clubs, private corporate facilities, tennis and racket clubs. There are tens of thousands of YMCAs and YWCAs that offer equipment and classes. There are Pilates studios and yoga studios. Hotels boast fitness centers, ranging from solitary rooms to sumptuous spas; cruise ships compete for bragging rights. There are women's-only clubs, such as Curves, and hard-core bodybuilding gyms. There are bare-bones storefronts without showers and lockers—and luxury retreats where treadmills and the newest resistance machines seem the merest afterthought.

Not so long ago the landscape looked very different. In the sixties and on into following decade, those who worked out did so in gyms that were small, with limited facilities and crude equipment. Vic Tanny and Jack LaLanne had pioneered the idea of upscale clubs as social gathering places, but they were few and far between. Ray Wilson had promoted clubs as spas, but mostly clubs were still gyms, dark, sweaty places that appealed only to hard-core weight lifters and musclemen. Bodybuilding appealed to a rabid but marginalized population.

Elsewhere, fitness enthusiasts were highly segmented. Personal training was fine for the rich and famous, but few had the clout or cash to hire a body butler. Millions of Americans had become converts to running, but many did little else. Beyond a cheery wave on the jogging path, the sexes rarely mixed. Simmons, like the buff stars who led dawn workouts on white-sand beaches, aimed his appeal at women who wanted to feel good and drop their dress size. The aerobic divas, the likes of Sorenson, Missett, and Fonda, had broader ambitions, but they, too, targeted women. Not many guys were lacing up Freestyle ballet slippers to join a Reebok step class. But men, too, were beginning to feel the urge to get in shape. In the early eighties, the first baby boomers were reaching their forties, and not all were pleased with what they faced in the mirror. Some had started to run to preserve the trim frames they remembered from decades past. Many had no idea what to do and no place to go—until the advent of health clubs.

Curious as it seems, health clubs—and in particular the big multiuse fitness facility—got their start with the spurt of interest in racket sports. In 1970 there were almost no indoor tennis courts. In New York City year-round players had to contend with the hardwood floor and dim lighting at a couple of armories. There was a converted airplane hangar in Seattle, an oil exposition center in Tulsa, a grainery in Buffalo, New York. Chicago had nothing but a scattering of suburban courts, but in the city nothing. It was extremely frustrating for a tennis aficionado like Alan Schwartz. What was he supposed to do during the eight months a year of cold weather?

Schwartz had captained his Yale tennis team and owned numerous state and national titles, including the Chicago Father and Son Championship, which he won with his dad, Kevie, a successful chemist who had developed Tennis Turf, a surface that cushioned the body and promised a reliable ball bounce. When his father was diagnosed with cancer and given a year to live, Schwartz made up his mind to do something. "I wanted to build something we both loved," he said.

His plans were on the audacious side: fourteen courts in an industrial wasteland on Elston Avenue. There was nothing there but manufacturing. It was miles from downtown. Players, he was told, would never come at night — and certainly not women. Plus, no one had ever built a tennis facility from the ground up, nothing on this scale. Not surprisingly, seventeen banks turned him down. It took a prep-school classmate and maverick banker to finally loan the money.

Midtown — a name picked more out of optimism than reality — began turning an immediate profit. Though tennis courts took up a lot of space, they also held distinct advantages for club owners. With limited options members were willing to pay high fees to join and play. Owners could count on "stickiness" — if one member quit, often to leave the area, invariably his or her partners filled the gap with another. There was a high degree of commitment and member retention. Schwartz, for his part, turned out to be a bold innovator; once he had his project launched, there was no stopping him. He came up with a catchy three-week program, "Tennis in No Time," designed to turn "tryers into stayers and stayers into players." He featured lessons and beefed up his pro staff. He designed programs aimed at women, well before Title IX required equal participation of the sexes in college sports. Membership soared, and within a year and a half he refinanced — banks were lining up now — and expanded to eighteen courts.

The success of Midtown spurred a building spree of indoor tennis clubs, especially in cold-weather climates. Schwartz's company, the Tennis Corporation of America, expanded the franchise with more clubs in the Chicago area and also in Boston, Indiana, and Kansas City. The most ambitious opened in upstate New York in Rochester, home to Kodak, Xerox, and Bausch and Laumb. Its core was tennis, but it also offered a range of fitness activities that would come to include golf, pools, yoga, navy SEAL boot camp, and every conceivable social activity from poetry readings to concerts to stroller fitness classes for moms.

The idea of an indoor sports club with separate areas for fitness proved especially popular in Schwartz's hometown, Chicago. In a span of six years, 1970–76, three major clubs opened: the McClurg Court Sports Center, the Lakeshore Athletic Club (LSAC), and the Edens Athletic Club. When the 1979 blizzard collapsed the roof of the original LSAC on Fullerton Avenue, owner Jordan Kaiser rebuilt it as a "country club in the city," containing two pools, weight training, racquet courts, dining, spa services, and a 450-yard indoor track. It was the largest health club in America in terms of both square footage and membership, though it did not hold that title long. One year later, in 1980, a true behemoth took over the record books: the sprawling 450,000-square-foot East Bank Club along the Chicago River. It was an indoor tennis and racquet club but with plenty of room for pools and gym equipment. With its proximity to both the Merchandise Mart and the city's downtown, the Loop, it quickly became a magnet for affluent young professionals. Traders from the commodity markets flocked there, as well as the city's most prominent politicians, and soon its bustling bar and restaurants were bringing in fifty million dollars in annual revenue.

Tennis was not the only sport in which men and women batted balls with rackets. In the late 1960s, in Milwaukee, Wisconsin, the director of the Jewish Community Center, Larry Lederman, noticed that his handball courts were being used more for "paddle racquets" than by the hard-core gloved players. He took the cue and launched an entirely new court game: racquetball. Rules were established and a governing body incorporated. More than three million players became converts to the game, and in 1974 the National Court Club Association was formed to represent the hundreds of racquetball clubs. As the craze began to peak in the late 1970s, however, club owners were looking at empty space and plummeting revenue. For many, the solution lay in converting the courts into fitness facilities.

Tennis courts, too, were beginning to catch the eye of entrepreneurs who wanted more bang for their buck. Though tennis continued to grow in popularity as a sport—the McEnroe-Connors battles amped up interest—indoor courts did not do much for the bottom line, especially when measured with the retail yardstick of revenue per square foot. A tennis court took up six thousand square feet; at three levels high it came to eighteen thousand cubic feet. In that same space an ambitious developer could carve out a basketball court, an exercise floor, even an indoor pool. The blueprint for this transformation belongs to Dale Dibble, often credited with fathering the multisports megaplex.

Dibble, an industrial designer and air force pilot who flew weather planes into hurricanes, had built a four-court indoor tennis club in Haverhill, Massachusetts, called Cedardale. With just two hundred members, the club produced modest revenue at best, and he added a small fitness facility. Then he added more—and more. By the time he and his partners were finished, they had a 175,000-square-foot multipurpose sports complex with outdoor ball fields and miniature golf courses. He set up a senior center, arranged corporate outings, started clubs within a club. Memberships soared, ultimately reaching eighty-five hundred, but Dibble was more than a numbers man. He was an organizational visionary, who pioneered the use of computers and club-management software. He put a major emphasis on staff incentives. Most important to fellow entrepreneurs, he readily shared what he had done, pleased to divulge all the details of his business model, and became a founding father of the club industry's trade association, the International Racquet and Sports Association. In recognition of his generosity and leadership, IRSA named its highest honor, the Distinguished Service Award, after Dibble. "Traveling to his club, Cedardale, and talking to its impresario was like making a pilgrimage to Mecca," said John McCarthy, the longtime executive director of IRSA, on the occasion of Dibble's death in 2010. "[He] developed the prototype and proved the viability of the indoor-outdoor, four seasons, multipurpose athletic club. He was the undisputed leader of the health club industry."

The new, bigger, and more diverse clubs changed the demographic of membership. Earlier gyms had been so space constricted that they allowed for only one locker room, leading to alternate men's and women's days. Now both sexes could come in at the same time, which enhanced a club's social buzz. In the old days most gyms were places to exercise. If you talked with another member, the conversation was about sets and routines and technique. With the start of the multisport complex, men—and women—came for different activities. They lingered; they chatted; they met new members. Women stopped by after leaving the kids at school or day care. Men (and women) dropped in for an after-work beer or to socialize at the juice bar.

Clubs were no longer just a place to build muscle (though it did not hurt to show off a little). Clubs had evolved into fitness-plus facilities. They had become, in the memorable term of Ray Oldenburg, a new "third place," a way station between home and office. In his 1989 book, *The Great Good Place*, Oldenburg had argued that such places were key posts for social interaction and the promotion of public activity. Clubs were growing to suit that need.

They were growing to suit another need, too, and it took shape, as did so many fitness trends, in body-conscious California. There, where physicality was all, the exercise floor suddenly crackled with a different kind of excitement. With its combustible mix of hard-body trainers and gorgeous models and actresses in crotch-hugging unitards, clubs like the Sports Connection in Los Angeles made singles bars look like gin-rummy parties. It was all immortalized in the 1985 movie *Perfect*, costarring John Travolta as a *Rolling Stone* reporter and Jamie Lee Curtis as the world's wildest (and lewdest) aerobics instructor. The film, though a critical flop and laughably bad in places, trod an intriguing line in both celebrating and mocking the men-hungry women who worked out to improve their dating potential with "perfect" bodies. None seemed more pitiable than future *Saturday Night Live* star Laraine Newman, whom a trainer called "the most used piece of equipment in the gym." But the film's nod to a tut-tutting feminist consciousness as well as journalism—it was based on an actual *Rolling Stone* feature—lost out to the hip-grinding Curtis and a pulse-pounding disco soundtrack. Travolta, the dance king of earlier movies, eventually pocketed his tape recorder and joined the fun. In the end he got his girl, the feisty Curtis, and clubs scored a promotional coup as sexual pickup hangouts.

There was new equipment to try, too. The emergence of aerobics and the groundbreaking work of Cooper stirred interest in cardiovascular machines. In 1969 Tinturi, a Finnish company, had introduced the W1 Exercise Bike, which became the benchmark stationary cycle for home use, selling more than one million bikes. Soon other versions were appearing in clubs. In 1973 the company Trotter introduced a revolutionary, easy-to-use treadmill developed by founder Edwin Trotter. Two years later, in 1975, Edward Pauls, a cross-country ski enthusiast, came out with the Nordic Track Cross-Country Ski Machine—a whole new way to pump up the heart; by the mid-1980s sales reached fifteen million dollars. In the latter part of the decade, a stationary bike with swinging handlebars, the Schwinn Airdyne, offered both upper- and lower-body movement. The Stairmaster, first introduced in 1984, became the most popular piece of cardio equipment in the early 1990s. A platform with rotating steps, its speed could be adjusted to suit the most challenging lower-body workout. A more friendly machine, less agonizing on the thighs, appeared in 1995 with the Precor Elliptical Trainer, and it revolutionized the cardio workout. With its sliding footpads, it eliminated the harsh impact of running on a treadmill and the intense muscle stress that could accompany a Stairmaster session. Treadmills evolved, offering new electronic programs and more forgiving padding; by the end of the twentieth century treadmills had become the most popular piece of cardiovascular equipment.

The upper body got its own share of attention. The same company that introduced the Stairmaster followed it with the Gravitron, a sturdy platform with an adjustable footrest that made it easier to do dips, chin-ups, and pull-ups. Cybex, a company that produced sturdy, high-quality "physical therapy" equipment, began to steal market share from Nautilus. Hammer Strength, the business launched by Arthur Jones's son Gary, brought out the first of a line of machines that would eventually be marketed under its new moniker, Life Fitness — the same company that manufactured the Lifecycle.

Separately and together, all these factors added up to a tipping point for club growth. The "penetration rate" — consumer participation — had hovered between 5 and 8 percent in the early seventies; a decade later, by the eighties, that figure had jumped to 16 percent. Clubs were popping up everywhere — and in every conceivable format. The Club Corporation of America, founded in 1957 as a golf and country-club company, launched a new concept, the so-called City Athletic clubs, which offered indoor racquet sports as well as fitness facilities and upscale restaurants for their well-heeled members. Big companies, the likes of Kimberly-Clark, Honeywell, PepsiCo, Chase, and General Foods, started featuring onsite fitness centers. Another organization, Cardio Fitness, marketed directly to corporations and set up clubs in New York and Chicago. The targeted marketing to senior executives had an important trickle-down effect, populating the workout floor with any midlevel employee who wanted to impress his boss. It was also the first initiative to stress the bottom-line benefits of fitness. Fit employees saved on health care costs.

The explosion of clubs tended to highlight a new breed of pioneer — more businessman than muscleman. Gone were the days when exercise legends such as Jack LaLanne and Vic Tanny used their celebrity and gym clout to promote fitness to the masses. The last marquee name among bodybuilders, Joe Gold, returned to the business in 1970 when he founded the World Gym chain, which grew to another three hundred locations. But the times were changing. The old barnstorming days of club growth had favored the likes of the hard-charging Ray Wilson, who built his chains with little more than a telephone and a micromanagement style that relied on total control. That style was fast growing obsolete, yet there were still individuals who powered the industry, though their names rarely showed up in the popular media.

LAST OF THE WILD MEN

Among these none played a bigger role than Donahue Wildman, a man who harked back to the Tanny era but who used his marketing muscle to turn Bally into the largest club operator in the world. The last name, Wildman, suited him. Born in Los Angeles in 1933, the only son of a fire-and-brimstone Pentecostal preacher, he had an unruly childhood and took out his aggression on the football field—and on fellow toughs. Fistfights landed him in juvenile court. Facing a likely arson charge—for torching a decrepit set of stadium bleachers—he opted for Korea. Shipped directly to the front line as a combat medic in 1950, he barely survived a first-day ambush when most of his company was killed. "When I got off the boat back in the U.S.," he said, "I kissed the ground."

Home in California, he worked a variety of jobs, anything he could get: plastering walls during the day, selling life insurance at night and on weekends. He had become a workout enthusiast, packing pounds of muscle onto his thin but wiry frame, which he did obsessively at Vic Tanny's gym in Burbank. Club life was less formal then, and no one noticed that Wildman and his buddies had never signed up as members—or minded that Wildman spent half his time peddling life insurance to actual dues-paying members.

What people did notice were women, whom Tanny began to woo in 1955. "It was revolutionary," said Wildman. "There were almost no women in gyms then. There were only these slenderizer places with vibrator belts and rollers. The male members were hostile, so [Tanny] arranged to have the women come Mondays, Wednesdays, and Fridays, because most women didn't work at the time."

Wildman himself took a part-time job working weekends—"I figured it would give me time to sell more insurance"—then got offered a full-time job by the new general manager, Rudy Smith, and decided to concentrate on the health club business. Tanny's was flourishing then, "expanding left and right," as Wildman put it, and he quickly played a bigger and bigger role in the organization. He was put in charge of a new Tanny club in Westwood; ran it for a year; left to head up a sales training team; got offered the job of general manager by Smith, who became vice president of operations; supervised the opening of more clubs; and got sent to New York and Chicago to beef up Tanny's empire. He earned a reputation as a savvy salesman and fixer who never balked at mixing it up with competitors. When Ray Wilson opened an American Health Silhouette spa directly opposite Tanny club, Wildman thought it "pretty poor sportsmanship"—and went into action. He crossed the street to Wilson's club and told the employees it was about to close. "I told them we'd give them jobs, but if they didn't leave today, they'd never have the opportunity again. Within days the place was a ghost gym."

Another time, facing encroachment from more Wilson clubs, he and Smith sent out mimeographed forms to alert employees to a creditors' meeting. When the clubs closed, he and Smith showed up at the Beverly Hills Hilton in black armbands. "People thought one of Tanny's children had died. No, we told them, it's to mark the passing of American Health. It was open warfare."

Tanny was suffering—though not from a death in the family. A lot of the trouble came from the selling of lifetime memberships. Wildman thought he understood. "He just didn't have much faith in the business. People didn't want to work out, no matter how good a service you gave them. They were lazy. It didn't matter if you sold them lifetime memberships—they'd never use them anyway."

The FTC was not so forgiving. Complaints were filed, and eventually Tanny went into Chapter 11. Among the bankrupt clubs were a half dozen in Chicago, where Wildman was sent to sort things out. It was a tough situation—hostile members, skeptical financiers. To boost morale he changed the name to Chicago Health Clubs. He started an advertising campaign. A friend and next-door neighbor was Ron Popeil—budding king of infomercials for the smokeless ashtray and Veg-O-Matic—who put him in touch with what was then the world's biggest ad agency, J. Walter Thompson.

The resulting ad was not the first time health clubs advertised on television, but it heralded a new era that peddled fitness with sex. Wildman had seen a Jamaican tourism ad with a woman in a wet T-shirt wading out of the water and arranged a similar shoot for a cold morning on Chicago's Oak Street beach. "I thought it looked really bad. The sun was coming up behind her, all you could see was her long hair. But my dad always said, 'Better lucky than smart,' and everybody had this fantasy of what she looked like." Even better was the exaggerated swing of her hips — also not on the story board. The night before, the model had sprained an ankle ice-skating. "She was limping like crazy, and the limp made her look twice as sexy. It turned out the best commercial we ever did," said Wildman. "That ad hit the jackpot."

Wildman went on a streak. Everyone wanted to unload the Tanny clubs. He partnered with a Detroit club owner, Roy Zurkowski, who had three. He took over clubs in Cleveland and in Joliet, Illinois; he started women's clubs in Milwaukee. Tanny himself had decamped for Florida, where he opened two clubs and then called Wildman to run them. In a major move Wildman took on Jack LaLanne in California, tapping his old buddy Rudy Smith to run clubs in Orange County. "I was always very ambitious," he said. "I wanted to build a big chain. I wanted to be the largest health club operator in the world."

The fiasco of Tanny's demise, however, had given the words *health club* a bad association. Members had been greeted by padlocks on the door; investors were wary. Wildman's operation needed a fresh start — and a new name, and so he invented the Health and Tennis Corporation of America (HTCA). "It gave it a little sizzle; it suggested a business that had been around for a while, and the bankers went, 'Oh, yeah, tennis clubs — we like that.' Actually three of our clubs did have tennis courts — three out of maybe a hundred — so it wasn't a total fabrication."

Under the name HTCA, he took over smaller clubs and built new ones. Most were better designed with new amenities — including what Wildman claimed was the first whirlpool. With Zurkowski now a fifty-fifty partner, he cannibalized many of the most prominent chains — President's, Holiday Universal, Jack LaLanne European Health Spas, even New York's celebrity hangout, the Vertical Club. HTCA soon became the nation's largest fitness-club chain, just as Wildman had plotted, with mid-1980s revenues that approached a half-billion dollars. In 1981 Wildman had considered taking the company public to raise cash but instead opted to sell — to Bally, a subsidiary of Bally Manufacturing. "They made me an offer that was hard to refuse. Everyone has their price," he said.

The price was $72.4 million, a deal that promised much more if HTCA met specified earning levels. Zurkowski and Wildman were named, respectively, chairman and president of Bally, each receiving close to $2 million in compensation. With Bally cash—Bally Manufacturing had plenty, thanks to Pac-Man and its dominance in casino gambling games—HTCA soon doubled in size, building a string of clubs that broke new ground in size, opulence, and promotion. With Zurkowski's initiative, they tapped Hollywood celebrities to hype Bally on television, the likes of Cher, Lynda Carter, Farrah Fawcett, and even Arnold. "I would sign them before they went galactic," explained Zurkowski. "I couldn't afford them later."

Wildman left Bally in 1987, by which time Bally had well over four hundred clubs, more than 25 percent of the entire market. Its purchase of the HTCA had anchored a hugely promising foothold in the health club boom of the eighties, but the next decade started poorly. Its Holiday Health Clubs had to cough up $9.5 million to settle a class-action lawsuit that accused Bally of racial discrimination against African Americans; the Internal Revenue Service hit the company with a $29 million bill for back income taxes. In 1996 the company spun off Bally Total Fitness, and Lee Hillman took over as CEO, vowing expansion and profits. Under Hillman the company trimmed its portfolio of low-profit clubs, renovated other facilities, and built new ones that put a premium on space: more room for weights and cardio equipment, no more pools and basketball courts. It plumped up the bottom line with in-club stores that sold Bally apparel, vitamins, supplements, and energy bars. It inked a deal with Baywatch Productions to promote Bally on the hot TV show *Baywatch*, which taped one entire episode at a Bally club. It went on an acquisition spree, picking up Pinnacle Fitness and Gorilla Sports Club chains in California. By the end of the decade, Bally had regained its clout and was the world's largest club operator.

Other club chains were forming, too, and gathering size and clout. It was like the geologic era when continents formed and swallowed up smaller landmasses. One of the biggest, second only to Bally (and often rivaling it in revenue), was 24-Hour Fitness, the work of Mark Mastrov, whose business would become a dominating force in the twentieth century and beyond. A college athlete and fitness enthusiast, Mastrov started part-time work at a small Oakland gym in exchange for free membership. He learned how gyms ran, focused on software, and had a revelation when he stayed past midnight and had to "flip the keys to the janitor crew. They had to open again in a couple of hours to be there for the graveyard shift. We'd never thought about all the people who worked in hospitals and groceries and factories. We never thought about the police and fire departments. That's what started the 24-hour strategy."

He became a gym manager, borrowed fifteen thousand dollars from his grandmother to buy a piece of the company, took over a group of Nautilus Health Spas, and added the "24-Hour" name. Under the banner of 24-Hour Nautilus, he raised more capital, opened more clubs—and set his eyes on the big competition in Southern California, the irrepressible Ray Wilson and his sixty-eight-club Family Fitness chain. "He was an industry legend, a trendsetter; he had a will to win; he never took no for an answer," said Mastrov. "A lot of people feared him. He was determined to the point of being aggressive—and very controlling. He micromanaged every one of those clubs with different partners. It was an antiquated model at the time. I was more of a top-down manager. I wanted to bring all those partnerships into one room."

It helped that Mastrov landed a major infusion of capital, and he bought Family Fitness for ninety-five million dollars from Wilson, who was eager to avoid another "open war"—the kind he had suffered with Wildman. The deal was the basis of an enduring old guard–new guard friendship between Wilson and Mastrov, and it firmly established Mastrov as a major player in the club landscape. Beyond his deal-making smarts, one of his key innovations was the use of electronic funds transfer. Sophisticated with software, Mastrov arranged for members' monthly dues to be withdrawn every month from a checking account. The old model—the one that did in the likes of Tanny—had relied on the sale of lifetime memberships to raise capital. "It was hand to mouth. You used the cash to pay bills or grow. In the old days you didn't care. You knew they weren't coming back. A lot of people make commitments in life and find excuses or reasons to stop. But eventually you ran out of people to keep selling to. We wanted to run the business more intelligently."

Incorporating the word *Fitness* from Wilson's chain, the 24-Hour Fitness chain continued to grow, using television and star endorsers such as LA Laker star Magic Johnson, who approached Mastrov to partner in inner cities. Wildman and Wilson before him had built their empires with aggressive personal swagger — Mastrov was more a low-key numbers man who relied on a back-office business model. For any individual, however, he respected what it took to build a club chain. "This is a very difficult industry to grow to scale," he said. "It's difficult because it's so capital intensive. But it's a service industry, and there's also a sales component. There are a lot of components. You've got to change with the times, multitask, keep the team together. It takes a lot of emotion and energy. It's like an onion — you keep peeling it, then eventually you get to the core and you start to cry."

THE AGE OF ASSOCIATIONS

Mastrov did very well for himself. A series of consolidations left him atop the industry, a club capo for other entrepreneurs who wanted to grow their businesses. Stepping down with his partners from 24-Hour Fitness in 2008, he founded New Evolution Ventures, a global marketing powerhouse that steered smaller brands to prominence. Not the least of them would be Hard Candy Fitness, launched by Madonna.

In the wild eighties, however, building a brick-and-mortar facility still had a frontier feel, even as fitness itself was enjoying an unprecedented boom. A younger demographic, men and women in the eighteen-to-thirty-five age bracket, latched onto exercise as a means of looking good and feeling good. Propelled equally by vanity and the chance of finding a mate or spouse, these so-called early adapters were a boon to club owners. Another vital driver of growth was the tail end of the baby boomers, people approaching middle age who felt the sudden need to stay in shape. But club owners who wanted to tap this ready population had few available models. How exactly did clubs work? What were the rules of membership? Which machines made sense on the exercise floor? Did you need to install a whirlpool? How much did you invest in lockers? In towels? The more ambitious multisport entrepreneurs made their pilgrimage to Cedardale for the perceived wisdom of Dale Dibble; others simply winged it.

It was in this vacuum that the industry's first — and only — club association was formed. Its start in 1981 reflected the root of clubs in racquet sports. Named the International Racquet and Sports Association, it was formed from two previous organizations — the National Court Club Association and the National Indoor Tennis Association. In the mid-1990s it stuck the word *Health* into its name and became the International Health, Racquet, and Sportsclub Association (IHRSA).

In 1982 it hosted its first convention and trade show in Las Vegas and represented more than four hundred clubs. It would grow quickly, sponsoring important research to give club owners a better grip on their business; its trade show would become the industry's grand bazaar, a carnival of a marketplace where club owners and equipment vendors inked deals. In 2012 IHRSA represented ten thousand clubs in seventy countries.

IHRSA was formed to meet the needs of for-profit clubs, but the fitness boom had created other needs, too. As the impact of individual pioneers lessened, the role of organizations became a major factor in growth. Indeed, the eighties might well be dubbed the Age of Associations (or, for anyone hoping to monitor them, the Age of Acronyms). The previous decade had seen muscle workouts spread beyond the bodybuilding culture to be incorporated as strength training for sports, and in 1978 the National Strength Coaches Association (NSCA) was formed to serve coaches of high school, college, and professional teams. In the mid-1980s it introduced its first certification—certified strength and conditioning specialist (CSCS)—which would become an essential credential for trainers throughout the health club industry.

Heightened participation in sports figured large in the reenergized role of the American College of Sports Medicine. The ACSM had been around since the midfifties, when it was a clinic-based group that served hospital needs. Somewhat pedagogical and headed mostly by doctors with a focus on exercise physiology, it broadened its scope with the health-fitness boom of the seventies. In 1975 the excitement of running (and its risks) prompted the ACSM's first position statement on "prevention of injuries during distance running." It was roused to further passion by the passage of Title IX, which opened the floodgates for sports-minded girls and women. When a respected Chicago gynecologist received a burst of publicity for declaring that "women are not built for jogging," the ACSM was quick to refute the doctor with its first "opinion statement," declaring, "There exists no conclusive scientific or medical evidence that long-distance running is contraindicated for the healthy, trained female athlete."

The ACSM statement, according to the head coach of the women's Olympic track and field team, "will put to rest once and for all the idea that women distance runners will fall apart. Incredibly enough, people still believe it." It was thus a major coup for the ACSM, as well as women's advocacy groups, when the International Olympic Committee decided to introduce the women's marathon for the 1984 Olympics.

That same year, 1984, the ACSM opened its new national headquarters in Indianapolis, which vitalized the organization. In the three decades since, it has greatly expanded its influence in the areas of exercise research, testing, and certification.

Certification in the eighties scarcely existed. A large population had latched onto the excitement of aerobics, but it was something of a Wild West frontier. The demand for classes was a boon to instructors but also a challenge — there was the constant pressure to cook up new routines. Even those leading branded programs, such as Jazzercise or Dance Aerobics, could be overnight converts with bare-bones training. Certainly, that was the view of one aerobics teacher, a recent graduate from San Diego State and phys-ed major, who came home at night to complain to her fiancé, "Almost none of these teachers have any background in physical education or anatomy or exercise physiology. They're creating a business, but there's no guidance."

The woman was Kathie Davis — she would marry Peter Davis, a fellow San Diego State tennis player and business major. Her aerobics career was in high gear; out of college she had been hired by a woman to create choreography, started training instructors, launched her own company, and had classes packed with a hundred women. "People realized what fun they could have while they exercised. Best of all, you didn't have to be an athlete to participate," she enthused. But the chaotic state of the teaching profession gnawed at her; she and Peter had long plotted to go into business together. It was the perfect storm of motivation and need.

Two years after graduating, they cofounded the International Dance Exercise Association. For its first convention at San Diego's Holiday Inn in 1984, they anticipated a modest turnout of two hundred, tops; six hundred showed up, and another six hundred were turned away because the Davises had not booked enough rooms or convention space. The following year they started the American Council of Exercise as a spin-off of the IDEA Foundation, and it quickly became — and remains — the largest certifying body in the world.

IDEA itself would see its growth mushroom as it expanded its franchise to include personal trainers and other fitness instructors, eventually changing its name to the IDEA Health and Fitness Association. In 2003 it added the "Inspire the World" campaign to tackle the obesity epidemic; in 2006 it launched an "Inner Idea" brand to focus on a "mind-body" spirit philosophy. In August 2012 IDEA held its thirtieth-anniversary convention in San Diego with 350 sessions. Upwards of ten thousand people attended. "It was nothing short of incredible," gushed Davis the week after. "When we first started, gosh, it was Jacki Sorenson and Judi Missett. And look at it now—it's amazing. We led the charge; we told people there was a whole new thing happening and you, too, can become a personal trainer."

Jane Fonda appeared to accept IDEA's 2012 Jack LaLanne Lifetime Achievement Award. Urging a new commitment to the benefits of exercise, especially for the very young and old, she declared: "Getting people physically active touches on the most profound level. This is psychological work we're doing. It was Thomas Jefferson who said, 'Revolution begins with the muscle.' Who knew!"

FUN TIMES IN THE FITNESS STUDIO

Group exercise today is a staple of most large fitness clubs. For many, it is the attraction that powers membership and is a key component in securing member retention. Women—the vast majority of participants—come for a variety of reasons. They come for the camaraderie, to lose weight, to get in shape, to feel energized. In the more family-oriented clubs, they schedule classes after they have dropped their kids at a swim class or at a tennis lesson or in club day care. In the edgier clubs the classes draw younger women who want to try fun, sexy workouts that range from Zumba to pole dancing. Some are devoted to a particular instructor or join because they have heard of an exciting new class.

Women had been exercising to instructors for decades, though often remotely. As far back as the fifties, Bonnie Prudden sold tens of thousands of records whose directions women dutifully listened to on their phonographs. Others watched the encouraging ballet-slipped LaLanne on a black-and-white television. The workouts grew livelier when Richard Simmons started prancing around in striped shorts and gym top. Mostly it was calisthenics, and there were no groups to speak of—the group was likely an audience of one, a solitary mom doing sit-ups or jumps on the living-room rug. All that began to change with the rise of aerobics and the classes led by Sorenson and Missett. Even these pioneering women, however, never matched the impact of Fonda and what she sold on videotapes. To many, it looked like a career option. "Fonda opened everyone's eyes," said Donna Cyrus, who heads up group exercise at the health club chain Crunch. "She had sex appeal and glamour. She said, 'Do these exercises and you can look like me!' She was an icon who merged the theater and entertainment business into fitness. A lot of people said, 'Wow, that's something I can do.' Up until that point it was all very sterile, very Jack LaLanne. It was something your mother watched."

Cyrus, like many who would go on to flourish in group fitness (or group exercise or, more commonly, "group ex"), came from the dance world. She had toyed with acting and had a bit part in *Saturday Night Fever* with Travolta as a girl walking down the street. The role, originally longer, was cut, and Cyrus continued with the challenge of making a living in dance. She struggled to find work in New York, spent a lot of time in classes, and then moved to Los Angeles where opportunities turned out to be even scarcer—until she found her inspiration in Fonda. "I realized, okay, no one's paying me to dance. But now I can stand up in front of a whole bunch of people and entertain a class. It was like a show. It was the hot thing to do."

Returning to the East Coast, she opened a small studio in Newport, Rhode Island, and then moved to Miami with her husband, who was in the restaurant business, and they opened Club Body Tech on South Beach. It was the early nineties, and South Beach was just becoming the nightlife mecca for fashionistas, glitterati, and anyone who wanted to gawk at Madonna and Cindy Crawford. Body Tech, one of the hottest clubs on the strip, caught the eye of Doug Levine, a former stockbroker who was prowling for new instructors to teach at the tiny basement aerobics studio he had opened on Manhattan's Lower East Side. He had called it Crunch and had a singular vision: to make workouts fun. Cyrus, he decided, should be his muse. "Doug wasn't a fitness person," said Cyrus. "He wanted to create a lifestyle brand. That's the DNA of Crunch: to offer inclusiveness, to give these people something they did outside the gym, not to lose weight or carve bodies like the covers of *Muscle and Fitness*. It was to be with like-minded people and create out-of-the-box workouts."

Cyrus delivered. At a time when other clubs were offering step classes and tame franchised routines, Crunch came up with Hip-Hop Aerobics featuring a live rapper and Cyked Yoga Cycling and Co-Ed Action Wrestling. Nothing was too crazy. With Cyrus at the helm, Crunch offered Cardio Strip-Tease and Stiletto Strength and Pole-Dancing. She recruited New York's most talked-about trainer, Jeff Martin, to brand his step class "Urban Rebounding" and had it debut at Crunch. She spotted the potential of a Miami dance workout called "Samba Tone" and told its originator, Alberto Perez, to "call it something no one could forget." They went through the alphabet to find a name that sounded like *samba* and landed on *Z*. Crunch was the first club to introduce Zumba.

There were classes led by drag queens (Abs, Thighs, and Gossip) and a Firefighter Workout that required dragging hoses up ten sets of risers. The chain, which would grow to dozens of clubs nationwide, lived up to its motto: "Crunch. No Judgments." It was a major turnaround for the industry and its sober focus on the benefits of exercise. Crunch was all about the ambience: nightclub lighting, walls painted violet and chartreuse green. It was all about selling the brand. No other clubs pushed the envelope quite like Crunch. California had established the buff-body culture; group fitness belonged to New York. "New York set the trend. Everyone watched New York," said Marcello Ehrhardt, a top instructor at Equinox and now head of group exercise at Lakeshore Sport and Fitness in Chicago. "It was incredible, very competitive. Whatever the studios were offering, members wanted more. They followed instructors like groupies. People were packed like sardines. It was a full-body workout; classes were *fun*. And if you joined a club, they were free!"

Instructors then were the rock stars of cardio, people like Martin and Molly Fox and Ehrhardt, whom *New York Magazine* would name the city's top instructor in its 2004 "Best of New York" roundup, citing his class Commotion! — a frenzied forty-five-minute circuit of mini trampolines, balls, steps, and jump ropes. "Class flies by and you end up drenched."

SPINNING GOLD

But the West Coast soon had its own phenomenon, and it, too, was transforming the aerobics studio, seemingly overnight. No was jumping around on the floor, however — in fact, no one was strictly on the floor. If you visited a club in the late eighties, you might have taken an experimental peek into the new dim-lit exercise studio and then just as quickly recoiled. The music was loud, intensely loud. In tight formation dozens of cyclists poured sweat as they hunched over handlebars, then stood on their pedals and went even faster, then slumped to gulp water. It looked like the heart-attack workout. It sounded, if you listened to the miked "presenter," like a blend of Zen Buddhism and Zig Ziglar, amped to the roof. It was Spinning, and if you were lucky enough to be in on the start, you had to have been following the wild ride of its inventor, Johnny Goldberg, a.k.a. Johnny G. "This is your life," he would begin with deceptive calm. "You have the power. Never stop believing in who you are. You are incredible. Ride your bike. Relax. Dig in. Let go. This is all about *you*. Find the champion within."

Few fitness crazes ever took off so fast. Within months, spinners were packing clubs in New York and LA. Celebrities on *The Tonight Show* touted its wonders. *Rolling Stone* and *Good Morning, America* called it "the fitness phenomenon of the nineties." By 1996 there were one thousand official Spinning centers. In 2003 the company trained its one hundred thousandth instructor.

Its flash of popularity notwithstanding, Goldberg did not invent Spinning overnight. He was born in South Africa in 1972. His father was a pharmacist and serious recreational athlete, who excelled in martial arts, swimming, and running; his mother was "heavily into yoga. We were a very health-conscious family." Biking figured large, and at age sixteen Goldberg took part in a five-hundred-mile cross–South Africa charity ride that forever fused his love of cycling with a spiritual quest for something beyond. "I embarked on that journey, and the bicycle became part of my life. There was a world of self-discovery I found on those long miles. I got the insight that there was more to bicycling than just peddling."

He earned a black belt in martial arts and came to America to pick up fitness ideas to bring back home. Instead, three days after he arrived, he was held up at gunpoint in Santa Monica and lost everything. Temporarily stranded, he decided to stay, ran into Joe Gold, got a free gym membership, and walked into a World Gym and asked for a job as trainer, promising to raise their gross 10 percent. He came up with a "two-for-one" membership offer that was so successful it turned into

World's global campaign. Recruited by a Hollywood manager, Sandy Geller, to privately train a few clients, he opened a tiny gym in Century City. Word spread, and the gym grew crowded with stars and singers. Burned-out and needing a break, he went back to his bicycle. He started racing, which led to triathlons, which led to longer races. In 1987 he tackled the grueling Race across America—and quit four hundred miles from the finish line in a state of hallucinatory exhaustion. "I think it must be like taking a birthing class and you think you have everything you need—until the labor pains kick in," he would later write. "Nothing could have prepared me for the spasms of my calves, the flesh ripping away from the seams of my bicycle shorts, while parts of myself drop along the road, skin and sweat and brain cells." It was a disaster, but also a lesson. "When an athlete learns to face adversity with maximum effort, there is a good chance to be victorious," he said. "All athletes must accept the fact that if you're not hurting, you're not going hard enough."

Thus emboldened, his training ramped up, he competed again in 1989, and finished the three-thousand-mile LA-to–New York endurance marathon in a mere ten days. How his racing led to Spinning depends on whom you ask. Most sources believe that he invented an exercise bike to stay in shape off-season. Johnny G.'s own version, a later perspective but perhaps closer to the truth, pins the invention on a loftier goal. He returned from the Race across America to a pregnant wife and the realization that "I had to do something with the rest of my life. The answer hit me: take everything I'd brought into making the mind and spirit and soul strong and translate it into the physical."

He made a stationary prototype of his racing bike in his garage. It featured a forty-pound flywheel connected directly to the pedals. There were no computer controls, no calorie counters, no gears—all that could be adjusted was a knob to change the resistance. He programmed a forty-minute class, envisioning hills and mountains and a like-minded group of spiritual strivers, and set it to music. Borrowing a term from cycling, he told his pals, "Come and catch a spin." One of those friends suggested that a great name for a class would be Spinning. "And that," said Johnny G., "was the beginning of the journey."

"Let go, get fit, live life, spin" was the workout mantra. A more graphic description appeared on promotional posters, which called the forty-minute class "part Tour de France, part yoga, and part 12th century torture chamber."

Johnny G. put it in more of a New Age context. "You could be next to an athlete, a model, it didn't matter," he said. "There was no competition, no winner or loser. For every human being, young and old, thin and fat, male and female, it was the opportunity to take leave of your body, to close your eyes and believe you were on that mountain, to find the champion in yourself, to throw your arms up and say, 'I can face these headwinds. I can get up that mountain.' It was empowering."

It was also a business smash. In 1991 Johnny G. teamed up with John Baudhuin, an avid cyclist and businessman, to refine the design and begin manufacture. In 1993 Crunch became the first club franchise to offer a Spinning class; in 1994 Mad Dogg Athletics was incorporated to trademark the Spinning name. Demand boomed for instructors, who were required to undergo a rigorous nine-month certification. In 1995 Schwinn, celebrating its one-hundredth anniversary, made a deal to build the Johnny G. Spinner, and the man it was named for, the half owner of Mad Dogg, became not just a legend but rich. He would officially retire in 2000, counting more than forty thousand instructors worldwide.

Among those captivated by Spinning in the midnineties was a young New Zealander, Phillip Mills, who was in Los Angeles on a track scholarship at UCLA. Back home his family had long been active in clubs and athletics. Mills's great-uncle had owned gyms in the twenties and thirties. His father, Les Mills, also a club owner, was a star of the Commonwealth Games and had won gold and silver medals in the discus and shot put. He had captained New Zealand's team in the 1960 Summer Olympics and held New Zealand's national shot-put record for forty-four years (ousted finally by sixteen-year-old Jacko Gill in 2011). In the 1990s he traded on his athletic renown to win election as the mayor of Auckland, New Zealand's largest city, and held the post for three terms.

Mills was extremely impressed by Spinning, largely because he had long labored after school in the family gyms, his main job "handing magazines to people on exercise bikes. All we had then were free weights and old exercises bikes that had wind resistance. It was so boring you couldn't keep people on those bikes for more than five minutes."

There were no magazines in the Spinning studio or in any of the other group-exercise studios, where Mills dropped by to work out and glean ideas to take home. What there was was a problem, Mills observed. Aerobics then was still wildly popular, but its very popularity had caused teachers to create more and more varied routines with more complex moves. "The simple reality," he said, "was the vast majority of teachers were not very good at it."

Even if they were good, it required a tremendous amount of work to create the choreography and find the right music. Ninety percent of teachers' time, as much as forty hours a week, was spent in devising routines. Why not, he reasoned, come up with a program that would tap the best choreographers, record the perfect music, revise the routines every few months – and sell it to health clubs?

The result was Les Mills International, a group-exercise franchise that Phillip spearheaded back home in New Zealand. "Every bit of research that's ever done confirms that people come to health clubs because they want results," said Mills. "They want to get in shape, lose weight, lose fat, get fitter. What the research doesn't tell you is why they go to health clubs instead of running around the block or working out in their living room. But there's a simple answer. Group exercise is the most powerful way to motivate people. You've got a teacher, music, crowd imaging, fun choreography – that's the key, that's what it's all about."

As of 2012 Les Mills had certified ninety thousand instructors in eighty countries. In the United States more than three thousand facilities leased its programs. The "jewel in the crown," as its promotional material puts it, is Les Mills BodyPump, a thumping, knock-off-the-pounds class currently offered in 12,700 clubs around the world.

HOME ALONE

Group exercise was all about camaraderie and energized bonding. But not everyone wanted to climb in a car and drive to a gym to sweat with strangers, particularly if your workout was aimed at building muscle. For those who could afford them, home gyms were an appealing alternative. Movie moguls and Hollywood stars preferred the privacy of a well-appointed basement or in-house facility. If you had a trainer, they showed up at your door. Nobody gawked on the exercise floor or slipped you a business card. The less famous had other reasons to guard their privacy. Clubs could be intimidating places, especially for those who were not already in gym-worthy shape. For all the lip service clubs paid to being inclusive and welcoming everyone, the majority of members came ready-made athletic and trim. Even prospective members in decent shape might feel the pressure to pump up in private before they approached the weight bench.

There was also the expense. There were the initiation fees and the monthly dues and the attendant guilt when one failed to show up on a regular basis. There was the inconvenience, the wasted time commuting. Granted, a home gym did not come cheap. Home machines — treadmills, ellipticals — cost a lot less than the high-end durable health club–quality machines, which had to withstand the stress of heavy use. But the price still ran high. Add a multipurpose workout station, such as the Universal or Magnum, and the cost could reach fifteen or twenty thousand dollars. But who said you needed an entire gym? Wasn't there plenty you could accomplish with one of those devices advertised on television?

Jake Steinfeld got into the home-equipment business in 1993 when, as he put it, he was "getting kind of bored doing fitness shows. I'd run out of things to do with a broomstick that were legal." A friend suggested the infomercial market, and he visited the offices of Diversified Products in Opelika, Alabama, with what he now says were serious doubts. "Infomercials? All I knew was the guys with funny sweaters selling vegetable slicers. Back then it was, 'You're on cable? Please don't sit in this restaurant.'"

He was in an executive's office when he spotted a machine in the corner. "I said, 'What's that?' He said, 'Nothing.' I said, 'Bring it over.' And I thought, 'I kind of like it.' If you could do leg presses and work your chest, maybe turn it around and work the triceps and back . . . do sit-ups . . . use those resistance bands . . ."

The first Firmflex infomercial aired in 1992. The results are up on the wall of Steinfeld's Los Angeles conference room, where a framed certificate reads: "Firmflex: Over 800,000 sold!" Ringing the room are other awards: "Cardio Cruiser: Over half a million sold!" and "Bun & Thigh Rocker: Over one million sold!" and "Ab & Back Plus: Infomercial of the Year!" He attributes his success to the trust he instills in the viewer — and to the product. "A little expensive, because it's not papier-mâché. God forbid you should sit on the product and get hurt. The manufacture is as good as it gets. Everything we do is sustained with science."

The same could not be said for other contraptions that promised miracle results and folded under the bed at night. Even Bowflex, the hugely successful standing apparatus from Nautilus, ran into trouble after dozens of purchasers reported injuries to the back, neck, and head when the machine's seat or backboard bench collapsed. In response to complaints from the Consumer Product Safety Commission, Bowflex issued a voluntary recall of 420,000 machines early in 2004; it withdrew another 680,000 toward the end of the year.

The Federal Trade Commission also fielded complaints, though few came directly from consumers. Mostly, it was competitors or advocacy groups that alerted the FTC, which then went after the miscreants. Even then few cases warranted review, though when it did investigate, the FTC tended to be blunt in its rulings. In 1992 a "cease and desist" order was issued against two Ohio companies that marketed the Gut Buster. The language should serve as a caution to anyone hoping for a quick exercise fix. Contrary to claims, the FTC found the Gut Buster did not:

A. Significantly flatten or trim the user's stomach;
B. Strengthen or tone the user's stomach or abdominal muscles sufficiently to significantly improve the user's waistline;
C. Burn or reduce stomach fat;
D. Achieve any of the effects described in subparagraph A through C above with a daily regimen of five minutes of use; or
E. Achieve stomach exercising or strengthening effects superior to those of ordinary sit-ups.

It further found that the Gut Buster could "pose a risk of injury to user from snapping or breaking of the product's spring or other parts" and ordered the companies to disclose these dangers in any future ads.

The FTC was busy again in the late 1990s when a series of Electronic Abdominal Exercise Belts ran nonstop on late-night infomercials. In its 2002 ruling against a trio of marketers, FTC chairman Timothy J. Muris issued this stern warning: "For years, marketers of diet and exercise products have been preying on overweight, out-of-shape consumers by hawking false hope in a pill, false hope in a bottle, and, now, in a belt. Unfortunately," he declared, "there are no magic pills, potions or pulsators for losing weight and getting into shape. The only winning combination is changing your diet and exercise."

The FTC then set up an "ab belts hotline," announcing that such "gadgets won't provide Six-Pack Abs," and provided these tips to consumers:

> Ignore claims that an exercise machine or device can provide long-lasting, easy "no-sweat" results in a short time. You can't get the benefits of exercise unless you exercise.
>
> Read the ad's fine print. The advertised results may be based on more than just using a machine; it also may be based on restricting calories.
>
> Be skeptical of testimonials and before-and-after pictures from "satisfied" customers. Their experiences may not be typical.

Steinfeld, the infomercial king, has never been sued by the FTC, though he did offer his own alert: "You got to use the stuff. It can't sit in your garage or hang on a door. It's like a book. If you don't read the book, how do you get the knowledge?"

CHAPTER 8

Fitness Today

Clubs spread—and consolidate; shifting fads and trends; the enduring power of yoga; the legends survive, despite crises and scandal

CLUBS: SURVIVAL OF THE FITTEST

As the world entered the second decade of the twenty-first century, much had shifted in the club industry. More than half the clubs that belonged to IHRSA were now outside the United States, with notable growth in China, Japan, Latin America, Australia, and South Africa. In the early days of club growth, much of the expansion derived from large chains. In 2012 the top-ten club companies represented less than 4 percent of all facilities.

There were, nevertheless, a handful of dominating players. Atop the list was 24-Hour Fitness, the privately held fitness chain with more than four hundred clubs and an estimated $1.5 billion in revenue. It counted more than three million members and about twenty thousand employees. Financier Theodore J. Forstmann bought the chain in 2005 from Mark Mastrov for $1.6 billion and relied on high-profile marketing strategies to bolster growth; the brand continued to be promoted by celebrities and athletes and was a partner in the hit reality TV show *The Biggest Loser*. 24-Hour Fitness sponsored the US Olympic team in Beijing and repeated that role in the 2012 Olympics in London.

Not far behind in revenue was LA Fitness International, founded in 1984, and Life Time Fitness, Inc., which started in 1990. Life Time, headquartered in Minneapolis, expanded aggressively in 2011—revenues shot up 11 percent—much the work of CEO and president Bahram Akradi, a native of Iran who moved at age seventeen to Colorado Springs,

Colorado, where he began his business career selling memberships for Nautilus Fitness Centers. One of the industry's top entrepreneurs, he made his name in Minneapolis with U.S. Swim and Fitness, sold the club to Bally and continued to run it, then left and launched Life Time when his noncompete clause expired. Akradi was big on growth and big on grabbing media attention. In 2010 Life Time staged "The Ride of a Life Time with 1,000 Spinning Cycles in the Downtown Target Center"; the two-hour "class" set a new Guinness World Record (topping the old record of six hundred Spinners in Texas at another Life Time–hosted event), with Akradi on his headset pumping away in front.

Bally Total Fitness clocked in at number 5 in revenue rankings from *Club Industry*, less than a third the size of 24-Hour Fitness and with its revenues plummeting 15 percent in 2011. Prospects had looked good in the midnineties when Bally Entertainment spun off Bally Health and Tennis Corp. — Don Wildman's company — as Bally Total Fitness Holding Corp., and its new CEO, Lee Hillman, launched his aggressive five-year plan to make the company profitable. But the seeds of doom were already planted, as Bally became a victim of its own aggressive marketing and the same ethical lapses that sank Vic Tanny in the early days of club expansion. In the 1990s thousands of consumers complained they had been forced to renew their memberships, even though the contracts were supposedly nonbinding. Others cited deceptive ads and high-pressure sales tactics that tricked them into signing long-term memberships. In New York State alone, six hundred individuals contacted the office of Attorney General Eliot Spitzer, which won consumers $139,000 against the company and required Bally to pay more to future claimants. Spitzer's office also slapped the company with a $200,000 bill to cover costs of the investigation. Most important, it ordered a full-scale revision of Bally's sales methods, including severe penalties for personnel who violated the guidelines. "People joining health clubs expect trimmer bodies, not trimmer wallets," said Spitzer. "This agreement will help consumers negotiate the terms and conditions of their membership and get the most for their money."

More trouble awaited, some of it related to brand management. The purchase of Crunch turned into a flop when Bally folded Crunch into its own Gorilla franchise, failing to recognize the unique identity of Crunch. Increasingly, the company became a financial sinkhole. It defaulted on debt, lost its acting CEO (Hillman had left), and filed for Chapter 11 bankruptcy protection in 2007 and then again in 2008. It no sooner exited bankruptcy than it was hit with financial fraud charges by the Securities and Exchange Commission and a $14 million arbitration award over a contract dispute. It sold Crunch and Gorilla, and then more clubs to pay off debt and survive, including 171 clubs to LA Fitness in 2011. In 2012 the once-dominant brand was a shadow of its former self.

Several clubs did not make *Club Industry*'s "Top 100" list because they chose not to provide the magazine with revenue figures. These included Equinox and Planet Fitness, which represented opposite ends of the fitness spectrum. Equinox typified the high range with an average monthly membership fee of $125. It was an upscale urban brand that offered a full range of facilities, from pools and spa to studios and spacious workout floors; Planet Fitness charged members $10 a month for an efficient if sparten workout. Gold's Gym, which had a lock on serious strength-training members, likewise did not share revenue details but did report more than 700 company-owned or franchised clubs. Curves also skipped divulging data, though the *Wall Street Journal* estimated revenue at more than $75 million for 2010, which led *Club Industry* editors to tag it a "likely" candidate for its top 25.

New clubs appeared all the time, though most tended to be part of a franchise or were small studio operations. The barriers to launching a large independent club were considerable, requiring serious capital, marketing savvy, and experience in the industry. Multipurpose facilities were unique ventures that had to be rooted in a solid business model and also interface with consumers. Small mom-and-pop studios, however, proved a tempting proposition for solo entrepreneurs. Little capital outlay was required to rent space, and even the equipment could be leased.

Rick Caro, an industry analyst and IHRSA cofounder, believed the primary challenge for new club owners, especially those between the high and low ends, was identifying their clientele. In the end Caro felt many fell victim to compromise. "'I don't have a full gym, but I'll offer half. Not four courts but two. Check that box. Nice locker rooms but small. The tiniest sauna or steam room you've ever seen, but I've got one. Check that box. I've got child care and try to serve all ages, six weeks to seven years. Check that box.' They try to accomplish a lot in space that's not articulated," said Caro. "You can't be all things to all people."

Veteran and rookie club owners had a major resource at their disposal if they joined the industry's powerful trade association, IHRSA, headquartered in Boston with a full-time staff of fifty. It publishes a magazine, books, newsletters, and detailed trend reports; stages a trade show extravaganza at its annual convention; and funds a variety of research studies that supply members with industry directions and updates.

IHRSA has also been a potent lobbying force, battling in states and in the nation's capital to ensure the unimpeded growth of the industry. At its 2012 convention IHRSA president Joe Moore proudly ticked off IHRSA's accomplishments over the past twelve months, most aimed at defeating "burdensome regulations" and an "onslaught of legislation." These efforts included:

- fighting sales taxes
- stopping personal trainer licensure
- protecting automatic renewals
- battling against restrictive business regulations
- fighting for a level playing field against tax-exempt competition
- promoting national legislation and tax credits to increase the number of people exercising in health clubs

Sales taxes, estimated IHRSA, could jack up the cost of running a club by as much as $35,000 annually. It could cost owners another $30,000 if they were barred from automatically renewing member contracts ("Health clubs are primary targets along with alarm companies and cell phone companies"). Consumer advocates might question several of these initiatives, notably loosening personal-training "licensure" and "protecting" automatic renewals. But these were battles fought for club owners, not on behalf of members.

IHRSA, and clubs themselves, faced a possible new challenge from exercise programs that targeted consumers who never set foot in clubs. A Canadian franchise, Flirty Girl Fitness, had surprising success with streaming video for women who wanted to exercise in private. Placing cameras in its hottest group fitness classes – everything from Sexy Sculpt to Bikini Bootcamp – it sold the video live online or made it available on demand. The chain took an even bolder step in 2012 when it sought to host private parties and charity events at its Chicago locations. Whether this heralded a new opportunity for the industry—or a doomed example of chutzpah—remained to be seen.

FADS AND EXERCISE TRENDS

Only with the luxury of hindsight can one separate the enduring innovation from the hot product that flopped before the ink had dried on the patent papers. The archives of fitness are replete with strange inventions that never survived their hyped marketing. Back in the nineteenth century it was air-compressed dumbbells and harnessed vibrating belts. More contemporary machines that seemed destined for best-sellerdom turned into abject failures. The Nordic Track Skier, which promised a total-body workout, looked like a slam dunk when it premiered in 1988, and it sold big in the direct-response industry. It proved a disaster at clubs. "Pieces of equipment that require a lot of technique are rarely successful," said Chris Clawson, CEO of Life Fitness, the world's largest wholesaler of fitness equipment. "People don't have the patience to develop technique. With the Nordic Skier it was hard to coordinate the upper and lower body, everything got out of whack, the ski went flying, and the user felt ridiculous. People don't want to look foolish in a health club."

The Stair Climber, once a dominant fixture on the cardio floor, was more often relegated to a couple of spots by the back wall. The elliptical, on the other hand, was an instant home run when it was introduced in the late nineties and has remained a top seller. The start-stop action of the Stair Climber could never compete with the rotary motion of the elliptical and its benefit of inertial movement.

Machines, in general, change relatively slowly in clubs. New ones obviously cost a lot to develop, and savvy club owners are alert to issues that do not affect the consumer, namely, the price tag, the machine's durability, its ease of use, and the availability of replacement parts and ready servicing. Handheld equipment and assorted strength and core devices can enjoy a much shorter life cycle. Anyone wandering into a health club can find ropes, elastic straps, and contoured weights that simply were not there the month of a previous visit. While some seem invented yesterday, others have been plucked from the dustbin of history. The kettlebell, now ubiquitous on the handheld weight rack, is a relic of nineteenth-century Russia and the days of Sandow. Its proponents are quick to exclaim about the full-body swing that builds neglected muscle groups, its century of neglect shrugged off as poor marketing.

As an industry, the manufacture of gym and exercise equipment is "in the decline phase of its life cycle," reported IBISWorld. That was due largely to declining sales by smaller domestic operators and stiff competition from imported goods. It may also reflect a switch from machines that target a single muscle in favor of broader, more "functional" exercise that utilizes, say, twenty-five-pound "shaking" ropes or even the body's own weight and balance to achieve results. With limited advances in product design, IBISWorld concluded, "There will not be any new innovations that will transform the industry."

That sobering view has not discouraged any number of hopeful entrepreneurs, if the trade-show floor at the 2012 IHRSA convention was any indication. It was anyone's guess which products would be around next year, but the merchants were brimming with hope and hype. Kangojumps, a sort of springy boot ("Gotta Bounce!"), had the tummy-tight models springing around like, well, kangaroos. There was a recumbent exercise bike with a balance ball for a seat—the Ball Bike. "We believe in innovation, not variation," promised its developer. "No other piece of cardio equipment uses the ball." On another stage a woman in a sports bra and barely legal shorts flung what looked like a stuffed pot holder to the floor and then lunged to grab it and fling it again. There was Kettle Yoga (that would be yoga with kettlebells) and the Body Blade from Peak Pilates, a twisty bow-like contraption with flexible ends. A trampoline device—the Cardio-Tramp Rebounder & Jumpboard Plate Combo— promised a "bounce and burn" workout. There were immense carousel-like devices with gym-clad volunteers pulling at resistance bands. At one, the Queenex, a muscled spokesman led the group like a carnival barker: "Yes, get low, say it, Queenex! Keep your hips high, like burlesque, yes, oh, good! One, two, three, four, come back, yeah! Feel good? Say it, Queenex!"

At Les Mills, the megaforce in group exercise, crowds gathered to toast the revolutionary "Shape Bar" with free food and champagne. The breakthrough was promoted by Phillip Mills, who had flown in from New Zealand. "For twenty years gyms have used the same piece of equipment—the barbell. This is the *new* shape. Feel the handles. It looks *fantastic*. Here's Suzy and Deb to demonstrate." Even Mills, however, could not compete with the crowds who stopped to gape at the Zumbathon stage where frenzied dancers spun to the blast of salsa. "Get up, get up! Work it, work it! I got you, here we go! Squeeze, control, use your back. Rock, rock, rock!"

Zumba was a case study in the propulsive power of brand marketing. In the time it took Sorenson's aerobic dance to go from a handful of instructors to one hundred, Zumba went from zero to five hundred – in New York alone. Between 2008 and 2012 the number of Zumba students surged from one million to twelve million. Worldwide, it counted more than one hundred thousand instructors in 2012, and in its single decade on the planet it had sold more than ten million tapes and DVDs.

The phenomenon got its storied start by accident when Alberto Perez, a Colombian dance instructor, forgot the programmed music for his class and improvised with a personal hodgepodge of merengue and salsa songs. Perez, who spoke no English, decamped for Miami, where he met another Alberto, Alberto Perlman, a recovering dot-com casualty whose mom had raved about Zumba; Perlman brought in a business pal, Alberto Aghion (perhaps it should have been named "Albertumba!"), whose sister was a Zumba fan. The trio jettisoned early plans of selling videos with low-budget infomercials in favor of building an instructor base, a canny business model. Clubs got Zumba free, and the company, Zumba Fitness, derived its revenue from fees it charged instructors, who needed attend only an eight-hour training to be certified.

Group fitness crazes have a way of exploding and then just as quickly vanishing. Billy Blank's Tae Bo workout, combining tae kwon do and boxing, was huge in the 1990s; ten years later you could buy the tapes for a song on Amazon. Zumba, in 2012, showed few signs of abating. A venture capital group and an investment firm created Zumba Fitness, LLC, pegging its worth at more than a half-billion dollars.

If the company maintained its momentum, the palpable reason was Zumba's touting the social quotient of exercise. "[People] love the red-hot energy, they love the results, but it's the thrill of friendship that keeps them coming back week after week," promised Zumba's slick promo brochure. That same appeal prompted IHRSA to name "Social Exercise" as number 4 in its "Top Health Club Trends" for 2012, declaring: "Again this year, Latin dance and nightclub-inspired workouts are appearing everywhere, generating a passion for aerobic dance not seen since the eighties." Citing its "fun" workout, the report noted the "great music" and "the group 'high' not offered by a lone treadmill."

IHRSA, one needed to remember, was the trade association of clubs. Of necessity and perhaps self-interest, it ignored trends that had little impact on its club membership. Escaping notice in its trend report, for instance, was the home exercise system P90X and its outspoken founder, Tony Horton.

P90X was more than a trend. It was (and likely still is) a phenomenon. The original P90 program and its endless spin-offs — P90X, the Power 90 Master Series, P90X One-on-One — was not the stuff for casual exercisers. It was a high-intensity, six-day-a-week "cross-training" method combining strength training, cardio, yoga, boxing, and stretching. The twelve-set DVD rotated through a series of "muscle confusion" workouts, all led by Horton and his gang of strapping teachers. What made it such a success was the appeal to the pain-and-perspiration set — and Horton.

A tough-as-nails drill sergeant, he mixed in doses of humor, honed during his brief career as a stand-up comic, and made no bones about his lack of fitness credentials. "Hey, George Bush became president. What was *his* experience? A lot of trainers are certified up the yin-yang and live in rent-controlled apartments out behind convalescent homes because they can't make a buck."

Horton earned his chops as a personal trainer with a client list that favored music stars (Billy Idol, Stevie Nicks, Bruce Springsteen), promoting speed and flexibility along with lean, rock-hard muscle. That same formula launched his successful 2001 Power 90 workout videos, under the corporate entity BeachBody, but it was not until 2005 that he hit the jackpot when he started flogging P90X nonstop on daytime cable. Three million people shelled out $140 for the twelve-DVD set, and, in its brief time on QVC, the sedate home-shopping network, Horton sold more than 135,000 units. When sales began slipping the company came up with a direct-sales scheme called Team BeachBody; friends sold the product to friends and pocketed a share of the revenues as well as commissions from other sellers they had recruited. Sales were expected to top $200 million in 2012. "If you look at direct marketing folks that aren't on television anymore," said Horton, "what they didn't do is work on building the brand."

The brand was big enough to warrant its own feature in *Men's Health*, the aspirant's bible of fitness that promised readers rock-hard abs, which it flaunted on every month's cover. The magazine also liked to stay honest with a nod toward journalism, and it tempered its glowing endorsement ("Unlike the garbage heap of other 'miracle' infomercial products, [P90X] can deliver results") with a page of *Men's Health* tips, sprinkled with Horton bromides.

The success of P90X and its ripped guru was part of a larger workout trend that grabbed attention in the first decade of the twenty-first century: boot camps. With their military edge and limited time frame, boot camps appealed to consumers looking for quick, tangible results. They were equally attractive to exercise rookies, who wanted to jump-start a habit, and hard-core veterans, who liked the macho intensity. Best of all, from the managerial perspective, trainers could run them in public parks; inclement weather only added to their reputation for toughness.

The prototype was Barry's Bootcamp, a West Hollywood staple that migrated east when trainers defected and competition grew stiff. It turned out no easier in New York where a boot-camp battle erupted between two rival marine-style programs, Pure Power and Warrior Fitness. It took a magistrate judge to settle charges of stolen business plans and operation models (two former Pure Power employees were ordered to pay $250,000). Triumphant, Warrior's Alexander Fell crowed, "What separates us, and differentiates us from Barry's and all others, is we are marines," which was not strictly true. A dozen other marines taught at New York boot camps, though Beast Boot Camp at Chelsea Piers had to make do with a former army sergeant.

Boot camps looked likely to grow in popularity as a hard-core segment of group fitness. At IDEA Davis was especially enthusiastic, seeing boot camps as the rare kind of program that attracted more men than women, the same demographic that signed up for workout-specific training aimed at competing in, say, triathlons. The value of targeted "functional" exercise was particularly appealing to aging baby boomers who had the time, money, and motivation to return to workouts with particular goals in mind. At the opposite end of the spectrum, so-called fusion classes that combined yoga, Pilates, and dance looked big in an IHRSA survey. For many, gym exhaustion had less to do with muscle fatigue than boredom, the endless repetition of the same workout. Classes that mixed up different routines tended to score big with members.

Personal trainers were another source of creative workouts, and the field enjoyed a surge in popularity during the first decade of the twenty-first century. Between 1999 and 2011, the number of Americans who hired a trainer jumped from 4 million to around 6.5 million. In part, this reflected a growth in what became known as "small-group training" (SGT). For the budget-conscious consumer impacted by the recession, the practice of getting "trained" in a cluster of five or six other club members took a load off the wallet. The popularity of SGT also benefited from the social benefits of working out with friends (or the prospect of acquiring new ones).

As the recession eased personal training resumed its growth as a career option, so much so that it began attracting a whole new group of professionals. "A Jobs Boom Built on Sweat in an Age of Belt-Tightening," trumpeted the *New York Times* in 2012. Health clubs were hiring; senior living facilities recruited teachers for the recreation room. There was even a growing market for parents who wanted their children trained. For trainers, the pay could be modest, especially at clubs that took 50 percent of the revenue, but the barriers to entry at least were low, especially if a trainer arranged for a diploma from an online certifier. "Once stereotyped as the domain of bodybuilders and gym devotees," wrote the *Times*' Catherine Rampell, "personal training is drawing the educated and uneducated; the young and old; men and women; the newly graduated, the recently laid-off and the long retired."

One place that will not be welcoming personal trainers, long retired or newly minted, is Planet Fitness. In 2011 its outspoken CEO, Mike Grondahl, announced that his chain was ending its hiring of one-on-one trainers. "Most of the people doing personal training are just renting friends," declared Grondahl. "For us to be selling personal training is a fraud and downright condescending to anyone who can breathe. Who the hell needs a friend for fifty bucks an hour?"

His decision and provocative comments were met with dismay, though not universally condemned. A few agreed the move fitted his business model; others found it an apt reflection of lowered standards. "I actually blame the big-box clubs and some of the certifying agencies," said Greg Justice, founder and creator of the Corporate Boot Camp System, "as they have set the bar so low that almost anyone qualifies as a trainer. Some of the certifying agencies are nothing more than 'puppy mills,' putting out as many trainers as they can, just to make a buck."

Hiring a personal trainer was not for everyone, especially those who balked at club fees during an economic downturn. The recession prompted untold numbers to give up club membership entirely—and replace it with a home workout. DVD sales enjoyed a jump in the five years leading up to 2012, with revenue climbing at an annual 11.2 percent. IBISWorld predicted an even higher growth pace for the next five years, promising annual revenues of close to three hundred million dollars. For budget-conscious consumers, a DVD or even a boxed set was a lot cheaper than shelling out money for a gym membership. Tracy Anderson, who sculpted the bodies of Madonna, Nicole Richie, and Jennifer Lopez, promoted her new DVDs for pregnant women with a T-shirt that read, "Staying in is the new going out in fitness." Stars and models drew the headlines, but the more significant growth came from noncelebrities and professional trainers, giving the industry added credence. Fitness spas and health resorts found DVDs a handy revenue stream and cunning way to sell the brand. In Arizona the luxury retreat Canyon Ranch put out its first DVD, *Canyon Ranch: Strong and Sculpted*, which shared shelf space with *Exhale: Core Fusion 30 Day Workout* from Exhale Spa.

Television pumped up sales. The reality-TV star Bethenny Frankel put out *Bethany's Skinnygirl Workout*, and, not surprisingly, the popularity of TV's *The Biggest Loser* made a video maven of its trainer, Jillian Michaels. Of all the genres yoga remained the top seller, thanks in part to the variety of styles, in part to the calm and serenity that home practice promised. Aging baby boomers, many urged by their physicians to exercise more, added to the market tapped by industry stalwarts like Kathy Smith. And none other than Jane Fonda returned with a DVD for aging adults.

Club membership maintained modest growth, with a new focus on efficiency and convenience. The recession prompted many to find jobs outside the nine-to-five structure, increasing the appeal of clubs that could accommodate an unorthodox work schedule and were open twenty-four hours a day. Anytime Fitness increased revenue 16 percent in 2011, close to the highest jump among major chains. Budget concerns were also a boon, if not a motivating force, behind the success of ultracheap membership at health club chains such as no-frills Planet Fitness. Other chains offered minimally staffed facilities in which members could check in and out with a key card. Finally, there was a new credibility attached to shorter workouts. Quick results with minimal effort had long been the staple of magazine covers that boasted "Bikini Butts in Ten Minutes a Day!," but new evidence suggested that long, arduous sessions were not always necessary. Many of the larger multipurpose facilities opened express locations. IHRSA pointed out that "most gyms and professionals are advising that shorter workouts of 30 minutes or less can be just as effective as longer ones." Gretchen Reynolds, the *New York Times* phys-ed columnist, had a big seller with her 2012 book, *20 Minutes or Less.*

There were, naturally, some types of exercise that simply could not be rushed.

YOGA

Yoga, of course, is much more than a trend, though it has seen a boom in popularity. In the United States alone an estimated twenty million people practice. From a virtually unheard-of obscure and scorned cult, yoga has swelled to include every lifestyle and demographic, and the range of disciplines is as varied as the people who practice it. For millions, yoga *is* their exercise. As a means to stay fit, it has had an uncommon impact on the growing attention to physical activity. Yet the reverse is also true. Yoga has itself benefited from the accelerated interest in fitness in America and might never have grown so popular were it not viewed as an exercise option. For years, for the better part of its century in America, yoga was largely a spiritual quest, focused on transcendence and escape from the body, or at least the union with a noncorporeal "other." It was often confused with meditation or linked to any number of New Age gurus and Eastern philosophies. That time, for better or worse, is largely gone. Today, most everyone who treks to class with a mat strapped over their shoulder does so in the belief that yoga makes them *feel* better, more fit and flexible, grounded and stronger.

For the record, yoga has been around a long time. Clay seals from the Indus Valley around 2500 BCE show figures in yoga-like poses. The most frequently cited early texts are the *Yoga Sutras*, circa 400 CE, which describe sitting as a path to enlightenment. Hatha yoga, the basis of postural yoga as we know it today, dates to the fifteenth century and the holy Hindu book *Hatha Yoga Pradipika*. The widespread study of yoga in the West is generally dated to 1931 with the publication of *Asanas*, Sanskrit for "Yoga poses," by Jagannath G. Gune, who had founded an ashram south of Bombay in 1924.

In fact, yoga in America was already well known then. Its enthusiasts ranged from Ralph Waldo Emerson and Henry James, who prized the relaxation of the "corpse" pose, to Mary Woodrow Wilson, the daughter of the president, whose practice took her to an ashram in India, where she ultimately died. Most significantly, it had a homegrown yogi, the so-called guru of Nyack, who held court on a sprawling two-hundred-acre estate two hours' drive north of New York City. The year that *Asanas* was published, 1931, future Pulitzer Prize winner Joseph Mitchell of the *New York World-Telegram* was dispatched to investigate the bizarre scene on the grounds, which included mansions, a new million-dollar clubhouse, a gym and theater, plus a trained herd of elephants. "A place of mystery," Mitchell wrote. "On summer afternoons townspeople crowd about the estate and look through the edges as the solemn students of Sanskrit go through their Oriental calisthenics."

The man who led the "calisthenics" was Dr. Pierre Bernard, otherwise known as "the Great Oom." Part mystic, part magician, part rogue, Bernard had made his first big splash in 1898 at an event sponsored by the San Francisco College of Suggestive Therapeutics, where he went into an "anesthetic trance" and had his lip sewn to his nose. Bernard (his given name was Perry Baker) would soon become a devotee of Tantrik yoga (as he spelled it), moved east, founded studios in Manhattan, and then arrived in Nyack, where he set up his luxury ashram. Yoga had adherents before Bernard—the likes of Thoreau, Emerson, and the Theosophists—but it was largely a mental discipline; Bernard embraced the whole body. Indeed, thanks to his focus on the sexual underpinnings of his practice, the union of male and female, he stirred up no shortage of scandal and often ran afoul of the law and its prudish constables. But he also attracted an A-list of notables, and the tentacles of his notoriety would touch people as varied as Ida Rolf, renowned as the originator of Rolfing; millionaire socialites, such as Anne Vanderbilt and Rebekah Harkness; and composer Leopold Stokowski, whose paramour, Greta Garbo, became a devotee. Bernard was an unabashed showman (Ringling Brothers borrowed his elephants for their circus) and swaggering egoist, but he was also a visionary who believed in the power of exercise as a path to the soul.

He never succeeded in putting his Tantrik yoga into the mainstream, nor did he much care to, and not long after his death in 1967 the Nyack estate was sold piecemeal by his wife, Claire DeVries, to pay off her debts. DeVries, in fact, went on to attract a considerable following in Hollywood, and Bernard's nephew, Theos Bernard, became a major force in disseminating yoga before he disappeared in Pakistan, leaving the Bernard name a compelling if largely forgotten footnote to yoga's birth in America.

The subsequent growth of yoga was an on-again, off-again affair. It gained a measure of notoriety thanks to the Beatles and their onetime guru, the Maharishi Mahesh Yogi, the quirky idol of a sixties counterculture entranced with all things Eastern. Another Hindu, Swami Satchidananda, delighted the massive crowd at Woodstock when he helicoptered in and sat in a lotus position flanked by devotees. Alan Ginsberg boosted the profile of yoga, as did Richard Alpert, who abandoned psychedelia and his onetime pal Timothy Leary for a different spiritual path and took the name Ram Dass.

Chanting and Krishna Consciousness, however, did little to promote yoga as a fitness practice. Nor did other charismatic gurus, most notoriously Swami Muktananda, whose celebrity and network of ashrams in the seventies ended in a flurry of charges of sexual abuse. But slowly yoga crept into the mainstream. In 1961 a hatha yoga teacher, Richard Hittleman, had taken over Jack LaLanne's morning slot on KTTV in Los Angeles and began airing *Yoga for Health*. Other TV stations followed suit. Daytime programs began spreading the word to Middle America. In 1975 the first issue of *Yoga Journal* was published. It paid scant heed to transcendence; instead, it was a practical how-to bible that emphasized vitality and health. Yoga could be therapeutic—and it was exercise, an obvious benefit in the practice of two influential yogis, Bikram Choudhury and Sri K. Pattabhi Jois, who had both arrived in the States in the early 1970s and whose arduous classes would help establish a new habit for Americans keen on physical activity.

Whoever gets credit for grounding the boom in yoga, there is little question how far it has come—both as a fitness pursuit and as a business.

Well over five *billion* dollars a year is spent on classes and products, including equipment, vacations and retreats, and media (DVDs, videos, and magazines). Beyond yoga's millions of active adherents, *Yoga Journal* estimated another twenty million are "extremely interested" in starting a practice, according to a 2011 survey in the magazine. *Yoga Journal* itself saw its paid circulation jump close to 6 percent in the year prior to its 2011 study.

Yoga, of course, is not a single monolithic entity. Its varied styles can have little in common beyond the use of a mat and the presence of a teacher at the front of the class. Its earliest practice, Tantric yoga, the loose basis for Bernard's Tantrik ideology, sought ecstatic union through sacred rites, notably sexuality, and came to be scorned for its excesses (vagabond beggar magicians who promoted incest and orgies). A dozen or so styles eventually evolved to take its place, many of them recent. Among the best known are Hatha, the gentlest form with its emphasis on postural work; Iyengar, a precise and formal practice, stressing alignment and held poses; Vinyasa, a fluid form that links body movement to breath; Ashtanga (introduced by Jois), a physically demanding style that ties breath to postural flow; and Bikram or "hot yoga" (Choudhury's contribution), the challenging routine of twenty-six poses in a steamy studio. What all these and assorted offshoots had in common was the almost evangelical faith among their practitioners that yoga provided a unique boon to health and fitness.

Anecdotal evidence and the swooning praise from students and teachers alike support this belief. So does the trim shape of many yogis, who are able to twist their limbs and bodies into the most unlikely poses or emerge from a rigorous ninety-minute workout with beatific smiles. Yet yoga, for much of the twentieth century, escaped the rigors of scientific scrutiny. In India Gune was the first to do detailed research on the physiological impact of yoga at his ashram in Mysore. The West had to wait another half century before a major study done at Duke University in the late 1980s looked at yoga's impact on fitness.

This, of course, was at the height of the aerobics surge in America, when Ken Cooper and Jim Fixx were touting the importance of cardiovascular exercise. Using the prevailing benchmark of VO2, announced by Cooper and supported in sports medicine and exercise physiology, the Duke researchers compared one hundred adults; one-third did Hatha yoga, one-third exercised on stationary bicycles, and a third did nothing. Disappointingly, at least to the yoga community, the control group—the exercisers—saw their VO2 jump 12 percent over a period of four months, whereas the yogis actually measured a small decline.

The results should not have come as a surprise; yoga did not seem the most likely exercise to pump up the blood. Most disciplines relied on static poses and, unlike a cardio workout, were aimed at calming the body's metabolic systems. But the yoga boosters soon had cause for optimism, at least when the practice incorporated the Sun Salutation. These vigorous connected poses, relatively recent in origin and central to the Ashtanga practice, required going from standing to bending to dropping to the floor and then standing again. If done rapidly, they could leave the heart pounding and the lungs gasping for air, which they did in a study from the University of California at Davis, released in 2001. VO2 rose 7 percent, not astounding but sufficient to gain widespread publicity. Cheered by the results, *Yoga Journal* assured its readers, "Yoga is all you need for a fit mind and body." In 2004 the magazine *Shape* told its readers they could dispense with "traditional cardio." To get in top shape they needed "nothing more than a yoga mat."

These rosy assessments did not sit well with everyone. In his 2011 book, *The Science of Yoga*, *New York Times* science journalist William J. Broad descried the Davis study for its many flaws (few participants, no control group, exaggerated claims) as well as the reassuring hype. "The Davis study and *Yoga Journal* articles quickly became the go-to-authorities around the globe for demonstrating that yoga alone was vigorous enough to meet the aerobic requirements," wrote Broad. "The door had opened a crack, and a blast of aggressive marketing shot through."

It remains uncertain how many take up yoga as a cardio workout; the number is likely low (with the exception of recent twists, such as "Power Yoga"). Many, however, continue to see it as exercise that, like any vigorous workout, will burn calories and lead to weight loss. If so, they may suffer the disillusionment faced by journalist and screenwriter Deborah Schoeneman, who wrote in a *New York Times* column: "I was an addict of ashtanga yoga for a decade. It made me strong. It made me feel superior to people who went to the gym. What it did not make me was skinny."

Schoeneman, who went to five and six classes a week, eventually cut back her schedule and began to work out with a personal trainer. Within months she had lost five pounds. Friends admired her "svelte frame" and "cut arms." Some asked for her secret. "'Less yoga,' I admitted sotto voce, with a note of sacrilege."

Her hushed confession touches on a problem with yoga. Loath to share qualms with an instructor, much less admit disappointment to fellow practitioners, many who do yoga continue it for the wrong reasons. Worse, they pursue it fanatically—and may risk injury. The possible damage resulting from yoga got a lot of attention with the publication of Broad's book and the *Times* excerpt of his detailed chapter on injuries. Merely sitting too long caused one man to lose feeling in his legs, resulting in near paralysis. A woman doing Seated Forward Bend fell asleep and suffered permanent nerve damage. Others had strokes, seizures, and heart attacks. The more challenging poses, inversions, caused fracture of the cervical vertebrae. Broad himself suffered a crippling back injury.

The spasm of publicity angered many yoga practitioners, who found Broad's litany of injury both irresponsible and alarmist. (He followed it a year later with an article that focused on men's particular susceptibility to injury, stirring up more debate.) Yoga entailed certain risks, as did any physical activity. Cyclists fell off bikes; runners died of strokes; gym exercisers injured backs and vertebrae. The danger, as in all these activities, often stemmed from people pushing themselves too far and too fast. Most responsible yoga instructors urged students to "go at your own pace; do only what's comfortable; don't pay attention to the person next to you." In fact, not everyone heeds that advice; many find it difficult to ignore their mat mates. They sneak peaks at their neighbor's Down Dog, they twist and bend beyond what their body tells them. And sometimes, rarely, they suffer the consequences.

It is generally agreed that the value of yoga far outweighs the risks, especially if one practices with a modicum of caution. The benefits can then be considerable, though weight loss is not high among them. Yoga has been shown to quell anxiety and lift depression. Its antistress utility figured big in Herbert Benson's best-selling 1975 book, *The Relaxation Response*. Mood enhancement is an almost universal plus for those who take yoga. It can begin before class, in the quiet unrolling of mats, in the focused calm that permeates a studio. "Our culture is so amped up, we're bombarded by input in our world," says Tom Quinn, a yoga teacher and cofounder of Yoga View in Chicago. "The yoga studio is a place to lie down, relax, and let go. Done correctly, it affects the nervous system and provides a fresh situation. Once you get used to that reset, nothing else works quite like yoga."

Yoga, it needs adding, was never entirely divorced from muscle building. Indeed, the two pursuits share an idiosynchratic past. As a means to get fit, yoga in the West has historically traced its roots to India and the migration of various gurus. In fact, several Indian yogis were heavily influenced by the "physical culture" movement in Europe and muscular Christianity. Sandow had a big impact on Hindu youth and nationalists, who looked for a new identity in a stronger physical body. K. V. Iyer, a famous Indian bodybuilder of the 1930s, credited yoga for his impressive physique: "Hata-Yoga, the ancient system of body-cult . . . had more to do in the making of me what I am to-day than all the bells, bars, steel-springs and strands I have used." But he was also a great admirer of Sandow, corresponded with Charles Atlas, and owed much to Bernarr Macfadden. His debt to Macfadden is obvious in an ad for his Physical Culture Correspondence School in Bangalore, picturing Iyer in a muscled pose under the bold-faced headline "Weakness Is Sin, Disease Is Death."

Nobody, however, better embodied the bridge between yoga and feats of strength than the remarkable Sri Chimnoy. Though never known exclusively as a yogi, Chimony's early spiritual path incorporated yoga principles, and he practiced meditation throughout his life. His example was startling proof that inner discipline coupled with exercise could lead to results that seemed almost unimaginable.

Born in 1931 in what is now Bangladesh, he was orphaned at age twelve and joined his older brothers at an ashram in Pondicherry, where he spent the next ten years. He came to America in 1964. Much has been made of his erudition (he lectured at Harvard, Yale, Oxford, and Cambridge) and precocious output (thousands of books, poems, and songs), but they were, if possible, eclipsed by his physical feats. A longtime mentor of Olympic gold medalist sprinter Carl Lewis, he became an avid long-distance runner and ran twenty-two marathons and five ultramarathons. When a knee injury forced him to hang up his track shoes at age fifty-four, he took up strength training. A strict vegetarian, he was never big—his weight hovered around 150—but he astonished audiences. He lifted anything and everything. Over the next two decades he raised platforms that held cars, planes, and elephants (one with Carl Lewis sitting atop). He raised and supported people overhead (eight thousand of them) with a single arm. At age sixty-seven he hefted twin three-hundred-pound dumbbells (guided by support tracks). In 2003, age eighty-two, he lifted Muhammad Ali and his wife overhead at the same time. The next year he lifted three hundred thousand pounds in a three-day solo marathon.

Throughout, he preached his gospel of interfaith harmony and earned many awards honoring his humanitarian work. He led meditations at the United Nations in New York. He attracted upwards of ten thousand students and the acclaim of world leaders. He had ongoing friendships with Nelson Mandela, Desmond Tutu, and Mikhail Gorbachev. His life was not without controversy. At least two disciples accused him of sexual misconduct, though Chimnoy claimed to be a committed celibate. Musician Carlos Santana, a devoted follower, eventually parted ways with Chimnoy and called him "vindictive." Denied firsthand observation, others have expressed skepticism about his astonishing feats of lifting; several doubters deem them shams. Nevertheless, few disputed the benediction of Gorbachev, who, on Chimnoy's death of a heart attack in 2007, called his passing "a loss for the world."

LEGAL SPEED BUMPS: TARNISHED LEGENDS?

The grousing (and possibly worse) that threatened to taint Chimnoy's legacy was not unique in the annals of fitness. It was, perhaps, understandable, if not exactly forgivable, that certain men (and they were always men) who lived outsized lives and forged their own agendas occasionally behaved badly. Mostly the infractions were mere sideshows, such as Hoffman's protracted feud with Weider, less harmful than a source of entertaining copy for bystanders. Even when disputes reached the courts, such as Hoffman's attempt to prove that Charles Atlas used weights, they did little to affect consumers.

Such was not the case with yogis. Most fitness pioneers, even the most celebrated, have had minimal impact on their fans' and followers' personal lives. There was an inherent distance built into the relationship, whether it was Jack LaLanne doing jumping jacks on television or Tony Horton leading classes on the beach. Most focused on the body and left it at that. Yoga teachers, however, often grafted a spiritual message onto their exercise, and the result could be a powerful aphrodisiac, for both student and teacher. Chimnoy was implicated only briefly (and, some would say, unfairly). The more flamboyant Choudhury, the founder of "hot yoga," was the focus of more long-lasting controversy when he defended yogi-student relationships in a magazine story, "Yogis Behaving Badly," explaining, "What happens when they say they will commit suicide unless you sleep with them? . . . Sometimes having an affair is the only way to save someone's life."

Swami Muktananda, who had hundreds of ashrams in the latter decades of the twentieth century, was accused by several female devotees of imposing unwanted intimacy. Others charged Swami Satchidananda, who gave the invocation at Woodstock, with molesting them; in 1997 a woman won a two-million-dollar suit against Swami Rama for initiating abuse and sex.

Charges of inappropriate sex recently claimed the most prominent American yogi, John Friend, the celebrated founder of Anusara yoga. Friend was a colorful Texan and early fan of Muktananda who had launched a freewheeling style of yoga based on "heart centering" and the "supreme consciousness," attracting more than six hundred thousand students. In 2011 a number of women in his inner circle revealed affairs with Friend, prompting dozens of teachers to demand he step down. Broad, the *Times*'s science reporter and author of *The Science of Yoga*, attempted to put the shock and surprise of these revelations into context. Yoga's roots in Tantric cults put a premium on the rapturous rewards of sex and yoga, said Broad. Even as a sanitized modern discipline, yoga could foster what he called "autoerotic bliss." But sex was not the only cause of Friend's downfall. He had also dabbled in witchy magic and had formed a wiccan coven that alienated many of his more somber and loyal teachers. They were further enraged when, to solve financial problems, he cut off their pensions without telling them. With his community in tatters, Friend went into a temporary retirement to think things over.

Not all the bad publicity that surfaced to tarnish fitness legends stemmed from issues of sexual misconduct or apparent arrogance. Joe Weider ran seriously afoul of the law in assorted actions, most aimed at the drugs and supplements he promoted in his magazines. In 1972 an investigation by U.S. postal inspectors charged Weider with inflating claims on Weider Formula 7, a supplement that promised consumers would "gain a pound per day" in muscle. Weider was forced to alter his marketing. Four years later, in 1976, a superior court judge required Weider to offer a refund to one hundred thousand California customers who had bought a "five-minute body shaper" based on false claims and misleading "before and after" photographs. The Federal Trade Commission stepped into the act in the 1980s, charging that ads for Weider's Anabolic Mega-Pak and Dynamic Life Essence were misleading; Weider agreed to pay a minimum of four hundred thousand dollars in refunds. In 2000 another FTC complaint targeted false claims for weight-loss products and cost the Weider organization another four hundred thousand dollars.

Other charges have also been leveled at Joe and Ben Weider, though few rose to the level of legal action. Alan Klein, a professor of sociology at Northeastern University, offered a sharp critique of the Weiders in his book *Little Big Men*, much of it aimed at the IFBB. In the view of Klein, the IFBB came to control an inordinate degree of power, sanctioning the most prestigious bodybuilding contests, and he identified competitors who complained that IFBB events were rigged to favor Weider loyalists. "Some have argued that the Weiders virtually admitted fixing the 1970 Mr. Olympia contest," wrote Klein. "Sergio Oliva, a black Cuban, had been, by popular reckoning, the largest and most muscular of the pack, yet Schwarzenegger had won. When queried about this selection of a winner, Joe Weider quipped, 'I put Sergio on the cover, I sell x magazines. I put Arnold on the cover, I sell 3x magazines.'"

Klein also cited instances of bodybuilders barred from placing ads in a Weider publication (he testified in court for one case), as well as drug companies whose ads might compete with Weider brands. In Klein's view the Weiders' near-monopolistic control of contests, magazines, and product led to a "feudal" fusion of economic and political clout that compromised the rules of fair play and democracy.

Weider's influence on the bodybuilding public has led to other charges that focused on subtler deceptions. Lou Schuler, a copy editor for *Muscle and Fitness* in the 1990s, praised Weider for rousing the couch potatoes of America to get up and exercise but worried about the example they followed. "His bodybuilding magazines were fundamentally dishonest about how the bodybuilders they promoted achieved their results," he wrote. "When you show a professional bodybuilder in contest condition and imply that the average reader can get similar results by following the bodybuilder's workout routine . . . well, that's horseshit and everyone knows it."

Trademark law proved a nettlesome issue as the pursuit of fitness grew more widespread in America, particularly when its popularity attached to certain brands or names. The disputes and repercussions were most telling in the drama that gripped Pilates. Joseph Pilates had died in 1965, leaving no designated heirs. Unofficially, his legacy was understood to belong to the Pilates Elders — the small group of students and instructors who could claim a direct connection to Uncle Joe or his training. Theoretically, anyone versed in the method could open a studio and brand it with the Pilates name, which is where the trouble started.

Among those teaching the method was the ambitious owner of the Manhattan-based Pilates Studio and franchises, Sean Gallagher, who had acquired the lapsed Pilates trademarks in the 1980s. Armed with the name and ample resources, he forced dozens of smaller competitors out of business or demanded they pay annual fees. In 1996 he sued Balanced Body, the largest manufacturer of Pilates equipment, claiming its use of the Pilates surname violated his trademark protection.

Prelitigation dragged on for four years, ending in a celebrated eleven-day trial in 2000. To prove that Pilates was an exercise method and not a brand name for goods or services, lawyers for Balanced Body pointed out its commonality had reached the pages of *Webster's Dictionary*. They called as witnesses several Pilates Elders who testified they had taught "Pilates" for years. Balanced Body argued that, like *aspirin*, the word *Pilates* had become so widespread that it had reached the status of "generic," meaning it was not entitled to trademark protection. In a ninety-three-page opinion, the U.S. district court agreed — and canceled Gallagher's trademark. "The idea that Gallagher owned 'Pilates' and that longtime teachers couldn't use it was ludicrous," declared Balanced Body's triumphant CEO, Ken Endelman. "The entire industry was being stifled, and the public was getting the short end of the stick. Someone had to stand up to this guy."

The historic opinion opened the floodgates. In Beverly Hills Ron Fletcher, who had originally referred to his training as "The Ron Fletcher Work" or "Fletcher Work," promptly renamed his studio "Fletcher Pilates." Thousands of studios without the benefit of a big-name hook benefited even more. In Ohio a major studio that has chronicled the life and work of its progenitor, added this truism: "Since the ruling, there has been an explosion of interest in mind-body disciplines and intelligent exercise options, which have finally catapulted Joseph Pilates' vision into a global phenomenon."

The debate over who was permitted to teach a particular fitness method got another legal airing in a yoga fracas. Bikram Choudhury, already in trouble for defending yogi-student relationships, went after another student, though not with any sexual intent. Instead, he tried to put him out of business. The man he sued was Greg Gumucio, who, after leaving his mentor, Choudhury, went on to offer "Traditional Hot Yoga" at a number of his Yoga to the People studios in New York City. Gumucio did not use Bikram's name, but he did follow Choudhury's strict sequence of twenty-six postures with the thermostat cranked to 105 degrees (and charged only eight dollars a class). In its decision the Performing Arts Division of the U.S. Copyright Office found that "exercises, including yoga exercises, do not constitute the subject matter that Congress intended to protect as choreography." Emboldened by the ruling, Gumucio sued Choudhury for reimbursement of legal fees.

THE LEGENDS LIVE ON — MORE BURNISHED THAN TARNISHED

The vast majority of lawsuits involving the fitness industry have had little to do with its name-brand pioneers. Clubs have sued other clubs for broken contracts or for noncompete violations. Members have sued clubs on a variety of grounds, ranging from attempts to enforce membership restrictions to injuries sustained in the club parking lot. In 2012 the member of one club sued both the club and the equipment manufacturer when a weight bench collapsed and he fractured his neck. Such instances are rare, and, with very few exceptions, none of the industry icons have had their names or reputations marred by suit or scandal. Even a dubious personality has done little to diminish the legends. For all their outrageous behavior, Macfadden, Hoffman, and even Dr. Pierre Bernard ("the Great Oom") were all the subject of largely celebratory biographies in the first decade of the twenty-first century. The worst that can be said of some is that, their life's work completed, they went quietly into the night. Charles Atlas, his headline days long over, died of a heart attack during a solo beach run in Florida.

Few who grew to prominence later, in the eighties, have gone quietly anywhere. Jackie Sorenson, the founder of Dance Aerobics, drifted from prominence with the collapse of her business but resumed pumping out DVDs as the founder of Jacki's, Inc., in DeLand, Florida (curiously, the same city where Arthur Jones came up with the Nautilus cam). She now creates 150 routines a year that are sold across the globe. The other queen of eighties aerobics, Judi Sheppard Missett, remains CEO of the company she started, Jazzercise; she choreographs new routines every ten weeks for the seventy-eight hundred franchised instructors. Jane Fonda took a long breather from the fitness business. In the years since she stopped producing workout books and tapes, she divorced Tom Hayden, married Ted Turner, converted to Christianity, and divorced Turner (whom she described as "needing a babysitter"). In what she liked to term the "third chapter" of her life, she became a fervent apostle of staying fit through exercise and healthy habits. "The difference between an older person who is active and one who isn't is enormous," she wrote in her latest book, *Prime Time*, and quoted an expert on aging, Dr. Walter Bortz, who said, "Fitness for the young person is an option, but for the older person it is an imperative."

Among the older surviving names, many continued their lifework well past their so-called physical prime, further evidence that the promise of fitness involved more than a passing effort at carving muscle or losing weight. Longevity may not be the test for a life well lived, but it is certainly the mark of robust health, especially when coupled with activity and productivity. By that standard many of the people profiled in this book have practiced what they preached and can tout its benefits.

Joseph Pilates, of course, is long dead, but a significant number of his most fervent followers—the revered "Pilates Elders"—survive. Most, like Ron Fletcher, went on to open their own studios and continue to be much acclaimed in both the fitness and the dance communities. Mary Bowen, who became a Jungian analyst, developed her Pilates Plus Psyche system to fuse movement with the unconscious and still works with students. Carola Trier, a professional dancer and acrobatic contortionist, studied anatomy and worked with rehab patients at Lenox Hill Hospital. Kathy Grant, a chorus girl at New York's famed Zanzibar Club, remains on the faculty of the Department of Dance at New York University. Eve Gentry cofounded the Dance Notation Bureau and was given the "Pioneer of Modern Dance" award by Bennington College in 1979. Romana Kryszanowska, the most celebrated if not the most fondly embraced of Pilates's acolytes, returned from fifteen years in Peru to take over the studio when Pilates's wife, Clara, retired. Clara herself, regarded by many as the foremost teacher, died in 1977 at the age of ninety-four.

Dr. Kenneth Cooper continues his work unabated in Texas. In 2006 he opened a second fitness center at Craig Ranch in McKinney, Texas, north of Dallas, a utopian community that blends a posh spa and medical clinics with condos for upscale home buyers. Never one to minimize his own impact, he proudly declares, "People thought stress testing was dangerous; it shouldn't be done. We went from a two-room office with 2 employees to a beautiful thirty-acre campus with 750 employees and a sixty-five-million-dollar budget." He talks in a feverish recitative, his message as seemingly urgent as when he first burst onto the scene in 1968. America needs to exercise; everyone needs to stay active; everyone needs to get "Cooperized." There are six basics to slowing the aging process, he reiterates. "Body index must be under 25, you must exercise at least one hundred fifty minutes a week. You must eliminate cigarette smoking completely, control alcohol, limit habit-forming drugs, and exercise proper nutrition." In 2008 Cooper received the Healthy Cup Award from the Harvard School of Public Health. "Dr. Cooper has been a pioneer in helping to change the social norm around exercise," said the school's dean, "making its preventive health affects accessible not only to athletes but to everyone."

The two pioneers who first brought fitness to television, Jack LaLanne and Bonnie Prudden, both born in 1913, never stopped working or promoting the benefits of exercise. Prudden eventually drifted from the public eye and moved to Tucson, Arizona, where she trademarked a method of reducing exercise pain, calling it Myotherapy, and started a clinic. It continues to operate with a half-dozen staff. She started her autobiography in 2002. "My sources tell me that my history and the history of Physical Fitness are inextricable. As I write this it is May of 2005 and I am halfway into my 91st year. [I] am just starting to write about my professional years beginning at age 39 in 1953."

LaLanne, a born showman and relentless self-promoter, got the lion's share of media attention. Unlike the musclemen of his era, he did not let age hasten his retirement from the public stage. The older he got, the more he concocted stunts to prove that anyone, no matter his years, could stay strong and fit. Each birthday he offered a new showstopper. At forty he swam the length of the Golden Gate Bridge underwater in frigid fifty-five-degree water, wearing 140 pounds of scuba gear, his progress marked by a red balloon bobbing along the surface. The following year he swam the two-plus miles from Alcatraz to San Francisco's Fisherman's Wharf—this time wearing handcuffs. Jumping out of the water, he threw himself to the ground and did thirty push-ups. At sixty he repeated the Alcatraz swim, this time handcuffed and shackled at the ankles—and towing a one-thousand-pound boat. Two years later, to celebrate the nation's bicentennial, he did a one-and-a-half-mile swim along Long Beach Harbor, handcuffed, shackled, and pulling thirteen boats (for the thirteen colonies), an armada estimated at twenty-five thousand pounds.

In 2010 his website followed the list of his accomplishments with the following quote: "It is most gratifying for me to see that everything that I was preaching and advocating for over 75 years has come to fruition. Then I was a crackpot and a charlatan, today I am an authority . . . and believe me, I can't die. It would ruin my image."

LaLanne and Prudden both died the following year, in 2011, months apart, aged ninety-eight.

Ben Weider died in 2008; his older brother, Joe, age ninety-three, died in 2013. Theirs, as noted, is a mixed legacy. Joe Weider's claim to kinship with the world's greatest marble sculptor, Michelangelo, was not entirely fanciful. He was the one who shaped and formed the Austrian Oak, though it is likely that Arnold would have found a way to dominate the world stage without his patronage and training. Weider did not invent his training techniques from scratch—he stood on the shoulders of many, as he readily acknowledged—but he did pioneer and formalize what would become key principles of bodybuilding. His publishing empire was a singular force in marketing the pumped-up body and, along with his and his brother Ben's global contest promotions, made it possible for musclemen to enjoy careers that promised money and fame. Whether too many paid a price by ingesting dangerous drugs and supplements, or whether wannabes were misled by the bulging specimens in his magazines, is not a question Weider chose to address. "The need for supplements varies from person to person," he wrote in an e-mail.

"Each person's body has different needs. Some people have a varied diet — others need help with supplements." His proudest achievement, he continued, "is making people aware of the importance of fitness and nutrition — how important it is to exercise and eat properly — and being fit mentally as well as physically."

In the latter part of his life, he contributed large amounts of money to philanthropy. The small amphitheater on Venice Beach where contests are still staged bears his name. Most notably, his two-million-dollar gift subsidized the Joe Weider Museum at the Stark Center at the University of Texas, which, under the supervision of Jan Todd and Terry Todd, is the world's greatest archive of bodybuilding lore and history.

Arnold, long retired from competitive bodybuilding, was elected governor of California in the special recall election to replace then governor Gray Davis in 2003 and then won a second term in 2006. His public image took a body blow in 2011 when he acknowledged a long-term relationship with a family housekeeper, admitted to fathering her child, and was soon sent packing by his wife, Maria Shriver. He chose not to run for a third term. He did, however, return to film in 2012 after an eight-year absence, starring in *The Expendables* with Sly Stallone, about whom he quipped: "Sly has killed 288 people. I've killed 289. We've always been really competitive. Who had the most muscles? Who had the most oil on their muscles?"

He penned the introduction to Weider's *Brothers of Iron*, praising his role as a trainer and mentor in business. Elsewhere, his name often surfaces when obituary writers seek comments for recently deceased fitness legends. When Weider died, he released a statement that read in part: "He was there for me constantly . . . and I will miss him dearly." On the occasion of Joe Gold's death in 2004, he was quoted: "Joe was a trusted friend and father figure and was instrumental in my training during my days as a bodybuilder. Gold's Gym was not only a training facility but it became a home to me. I will miss him as a dear friend of 36 years." He had similar words on the 2011 death of Roy Zurkowski, the cofounder of the HTCA with Donahue Wildman: "Roy was a great fitness leader," he said, "a great entrepreneur and a fantastic friend. We had a wonderful friendship and Maria and I were very sad to hear of his passing."

Wildman himself remains very much alive. He might easily have retired quietly with the comfy fortune he made from selling his business to Bally. He did the opposite. While still at Bally he had watched the first televised Hawaiian Ironman triathlon, touted as the ultimate physical challenge. The race lived up to its reputation, certainly for the women's leader, Julie Moss, who collapsed two hundred yards from the end of the marathon and then dragged herself and crawled to the finish line, where she sprawled in a puddle of urine while her eyes rolled back in her head. Watching the horrifying spectacle, Wildman told his wife, "Hey, there's this new sport I want to try."

In subsequent years Wildman completed nine Ironman triathlons. He biked three thousand miles cross-country in the Race across America challenge. He ran the New York and LA Marathons. Sailing, he won the Chicago Yacht Club's famed Mackinac Race. He paddled the entire chain of Hawaiian Islands on a surfboard with his new best pal, Laird Hamilton, the surfing legend, whom he had met while the two were snowboarding. Enticed by Hamilton to try tow surfing behind a jet ski in twenty-foot swells, he got slammed twice before giving it a third try. "It felt like a Mack truck hit me, and I went, 'Whoa, this is pretty good.'"

In his midseventies he periodically hosts journalists who dutifully train and then gasp to keep up with Wildman on his impossibly rugged ten-mile morning run through the Malibu hills. Three days a week he leads a two-hour punishing weight workout called the Circuit for a small cadre of friends and fellow masochists.

One friend, Ray Wilson, Wildman's long-ago rival in the "gym wars," is too infirm to travel much and visit Wildman, though they talk on the phone. Hobbled by back injuries he suffered during his early wrestling career, he remains as feisty and outspoken as ever with an uncanny memory for the minutiae of his long career and many close associates. He was especially moved by the death of his onetime business partner, Bob Delmonteque, in 2012: "Bob was a very loyal friend," he wrote in an e-mail, "and did a huge amount of good for the fitness industry. Like Jack LaLanne [he] was an inspiration to be around."

Several fitness pioneers, younger than Wilson and Wildman by decades, have had their work and lives abbreviated by health crises. Johnny G. was only fifty-three, at the height of his career, when he was diagnosed with a viral infection in his heart. The impact was devastating. Today he lives quietly in a sprawling ranch-style home near Santa Barbara set amid lush landscaped grounds. There is a pond beyond the patio. Lilting music drifts through the airy rooms that are appointed with Chinese art and Oriental screens. He exercises only in moderation, has a pacemaker, takes a lot of medication, and coils his body carefully on a low bolster cushion to talk to a visitor. Though he will never again be the wild exercise guru urging friends to come by and "catch a spin," he has not been idle. In 2010 he patented a new machine — the Krankcycle. It combines a pedaled bike with a vigorous rotary arm exercise, the only "upper-body aerobic workout," and has achieved modest penetration in the marketplace. He is most excited by his latest invention, the "Intrinity," which he promises will transform ideas of exercise. It is a device — a board, really — that allows its user to reach around and below. "I've changed the environment of exercise. I've removed the floor. I've created negative space." What the future holds, what he can hope for, what he always hoped to inspire in those who followed him is what Goldberg still calls "the joy of the journey."

Augie Nieto suffered a more debilitating tragedy, also in the prime of his career. The year was 2004, and the future looked bright. He had made a pile of money when, for the second time, he sold the rights to Life Fitness, the company he cofounded to manufacture the Lifecycle. An early sponsor of IRSA and a tireless advocate of global fitness, he traveled the world to promote the benefits of exercise. He took adventurous trips to Tibet, Nepal, and India, often with his family, which included three children and his wife, Lynne, the cheerleader from Claremont College. It was on one of these trips, water-skiing in Vietnam's Mekong Delta, that his arms went suddenly slack. He could barely pull himself from the water. A short time later he was diagnosed with amyotrophic lateral sclerosis, or ALS — Lou Gehrig's disease.

It was a grim and ironic fate for the man who had thrilled in his own physicality. The disease attacks the muscular system and is almost always fatal. There is no cure. Its deadly progression leaves the victim increasingly helpless, unable to move limbs, and, finally, unable to exert control over the basic functions of life. Two years after the diagnosis, in 2006, he was confined to a wheelchair. Lacking upper-body mobility, he could no longer eat unassisted. With Lynne alongside, a full-time helper had wheeled him into the living room of his California home in Corona del Mar with its spectacular view of the Pacific. His voice was little more than a whisper, though he had spoken at Harvard the week before — one of the last trips he would make — to preach his new gospel, "From Success to Significance." "I'm a huge believer in floating the boat," he said that morning. "If you can grow the market, everyone benefits; that's been my focus from day one. Instead of saying, 'I'm going to take food from my competitor,' I've preferred to bring more food to the table so we both can eat. I look for people who give versus get. That's my platform, and people listen to me. I have the ability to connect. I have a gift right now to see things that most people don't. I'm a dead man walking."

Six years later he was still alive, though he could no longer speak and rarely left his bed. But those diminished capacities had only fueled his desire to make a success of Augie's Quest — his mission to find a cure for ALS. Thousands of people, friends and strangers and admirers — among them then governor Schwarzenegger — had given time and money and support to join Nieto's crusade, which focused on stem-cell research. Subsidized by money he had raised, a promising drug was moving through clinical trials. As at every IHRSA convention, the 2012 gathering in Los Angeles featured a gala dinner that was a benefit for Augie's Quest. Defying the odds, Nieto managed to make an appearance in support of the vow he had made to his college alumni magazine. "I believe there's a cure," he told the reporter, "and I don't take no for an answer. This is no different from when I knocked on people's doors and tried to sell them a Lifecycle. I believed they needed it."

Richard Simmons, defying a different kind of odds, continues his own lifelong crusade, seemingly immune to the rolled eyes and innuendo of TV talk show hosts, on whose shows he was a reliable guest and camp clown. He did have his limits. On *Late Night with David Letterman*, he came dressed as a Thanksgiving turkey but then, after grabbing Letterman in a comic sexual hug, was sprayed with a fire extinguisher and suffered an acute asthma attack. Boycotting the show for six years, he returned to be victimized by another prank — an exploding steamer tray. He had a similar on-again, off-again relationship with radio shock jock Howard Stern in the 1990s, swore off being a guest after an excess of insults, and then returned in 2012. He was treated with more civility by Jay Leno.

He still leads classes. Three nights a week — "when Richard is in town," reads his website — he parks his black Range Rover in front of "Richard

Slimmons," his spacious studio off Santa Monica Boulevard. The cost of the hour-long workout is twelve dollars. No reservations, guests are invited to start lining up an hour before class starts. Cameras and cell-phone pictures are not permitted, though Simmons will pose if requested. The aerobics room can accommodate one hundred persons and is often filled to capacity, largely by women. On one particular evening Simmons sailed in only minutes before the 6:30 class, dressed in a black toga-like outfit with fake-gold jewelry banding his arms and a cloth cobra dangling from his neck. "Didn't you hear?" he exclaimed. "It's costume night!" He greeted half the guests by name, hugged everyone, and ran inside to crank up the music. The Sultan of Sweat was alive and well and making a buck.

CHAPTER 9

Why Exercise?

Tackling the obesity epidemic; what exactly does it mean to be fit? a challenging—and hopeful—future

WHAT IT MEANS TO BE FIT

It's easiest, of course, to identify what it means *not* to be fit. The facts are both everywhere and alarming. America is in the midst of an obesity epidemic. As recently as 1990 fewer than 10 percent of adults were obese; that figure has now doubled. In three states one-third of all adults are considered obese. Add those who are merely overweight (defined as having a body mass index between 25 and 29.9), and the number of Americans who weigh more than they should reaches six out of ten. Obesity is the primary risk factor in three leading causes of death and infirmity: it affects the muscular-skeletal system, it impacts the cardiovascular system, and it contributes to diabetes. Between 1997 and 2004 the incidence of diabetes saw a startling rise: the number of new cases jumped by 54 percent. More disturbing, a growing number of children are contracting obesity-linked diabetes. Type 2 diabetes, which used to be so rare in children it was called adult-onset diabetes, is afflicting increasing numbers of teens, many in low-income families. The duration of the disease greatly increases the risk of future problems.

Most experts agree that the twin causes of obesity are poor nutrition and lack of exercise. Advocates of healthier eating habits have made significant strides in reducing harmful food and promoting better choices. Fast-food franchises have cut back on fatty oils. There are more salads on the menu, less sugar and less sodium. The Food and Drug Administration continues to revise its food chart to prioritize fruits and vegetables. School lunch programs feature salads. There are fewer chemicals and preservatives in the cartons and cans at the supermarket. These successes, unfortunately, have yet to stem the habits of a culture addicted to sugar and grease and fast-food snacks. Nor, some argue, can nutrition alone reverse the trend. A long time ago Hippocrates, who should know, said, "Eating alone will not keep a man well; he must also take exercise."

Lynda Powell is the chairman of Preventive Medicine at Rush Medical Center in Chicago, and she could not agree more. "You can't work alone in the diet realm. We used to think that you dealt with obesity by getting people to eat less. Now there's more focus on physical activity to promote sustained change. If people are active, that moderates their energy intake and reaction to stress, which impacts caloric intake. People need to get up and move."

It is not an easy sell. What Bonnie Prudden lamented as "couch-potato-ism" has taken on frightening new dimensions in a world entranced with smartphones, laptops, and the Internet. Particularly for the young, ours has become a sedentary culture (again), with little excitement to rival what is available onscreen or in text. We no longer walk to bookstores (there are none) or even to the local video outlet (so much easier and cheaper to get our entertainment streaming online). Pizza and fifty-four-inch plasma TVs keep us rooted to the living-room sofa. In July 2012 *Newsweek* ran a cover story, "iCrazy," detailing the dimensions of the problem. Recent studies found that Americans slumped for five hours daily in front of the television, a habit that begins early, with the TV used to babysit toddlers. With jobs scarce during a recession, more of us work at home (or simply stay there), reducing the getting-to-work exercise. At home we move around less, further cutting back on what exercise physiologists call "light-intensity activity." First Lady Michelle Obama's "Let's Move!" campaign from the White House lawn played big on the nightly news, but how many heeded her advice?

Powell, for one, has identified a crucial obstacle. The people enrolled in her program are mostly older, average age fifty-two, and come for help with obesity through referrals from primary-care physicians or Rush advertising. But Powell believes the insights she has developed are applicable to people of any age and size; namely, we sabotage our best intentions by focusing on an end goal that is way too extreme, a bad American habit she calls "going from zero to one hundred." Those who launch into exercise programs with that ultimate goal in mind get frustrated, and when they do, "they rebound to couch potatoes."

Far better to think like the French, says Powell. French women live longer than any women in the world. French men come in second only to the Japanese. What ensures their longevity is not red wine or foie gras or chocolate – it is moderation. The women drink one to two glasses of wine – small glasses, stresses Powell – and always with meals. French men drink two to three glasses – with food. Powell spent a year in Paris at the Epidemiological Institute studying diet and exercise, but it is what she observed on the streets that changed her views. "If I saw a person running around a park, sweating, it was always an American. The French don't do that. They think our obsession with intensity is a joke. It's how they ridicule American culture."

Americans need to take smaller steps, argues Powell. Go from zero to ten, then twenty or thirty. Appreciate the side benefits of exercise. Enjoy what Powell calls the "immediate reenforcers. Take a walk, enjoy the fresh air or the uninterrupted quiet; find a walking companion and have a conversation." It is no accident that we term exercise a "workout." Physical activity, she stresses, should be enjoyable "and not part of the American work ethic."

It is worth quoting Jim Fixx who, way back in 1978, the year his first book was published, hailed running for benefits that included better health, better body shape, and better sex, but ended with this: "Most important, running is fun. Many of us have been brought up to feel that any physical effort must be made out of a sense of duty. The armed forces conditioning programs certainly make us feel that way, as do most physical training programs in our schools and, in the opinion of many, Kenneth Cooper's forbidding and joyless aerobics charts; you run so far in so many minutes simply to earn aerobics points. But if you miss the pleasure in running you miss its essence." He went on to extol the idyllic delights of his hour-long autumn run: the crisp air, bright-colored leaves swirling underfoot, rabbits and chipmunks that "scatter at the sound of my footsteps." He returned home "spent but exhilarated."

The notion of fun and uplift as a lure to first-time exercisers has figured only peripherally in the long history of fitness in America. The point of exercise, what so many early crusaders sold, was not the activity but the results. Muscles built confidence: on the beach, in the cookie-cutter offices of urban America, in the Cold War face-off with an intimidating enemy. As fitness osmosed into the popular culture, through movies, television, video, and mainstream magazines, the goals grew more diffuse. It was enough to look good, tone up the body, lose a few pounds—and enjoy the new multisports clubs that offered carrot shakes and a hot-tub soak after a turn on the Nautilus. Then, just when America was beginning to relax, along came the "joyless" Ken Cooper, and fitness was no longer a casual option. Suddenly, it became a matter of life and death, a prerequisite of health.

Health was easier to define than fitness. Broadly speaking, it meant minimizing the risk factors that contributed to premature death. Sitting around too much was unhealthy. Watching hours of daytime television or confusing sunlight with the glow from a laptop screen was unhealthy. The body required exercise, whether it was walking, gardening, or scattering the chipmunks on an autumn run.

But what exactly was fitness? For many, it meant functional fitness—the ability to tackle a particular sport or activity and perform at a high level. Jim Fixx was functionally fit—but he was not healthy. Whether running prolonged his life or hastened its end was a meaningless debate; the more relevant fact was that he should have seen a doctor. A number of history's most impressive weight lifters and bodybuilders were functionally fit; they lifted piles of iron or posed with bulging veins in muscle magazines. But many were far from healthy, especially if they pumped up their bodies with drugs and supplements whose corrosive effect caused irreparable damage to their hearts.

Overall fitness remains a more elusive concept. Its definition still owes much to Cooper, whose *Aerobics* focused attention on cardiovascular activity. The measurement, VO2 max, stood for the amount of oxygen the heart and lungs could pump and distribute to working muscles. Countless studies have confirmed its primacy as a clue to health. Citing "a growing body of science," *New York Times* phys-ed columnist Gretchen Reynolds declared that "aerobic fitness may be the single most important determinant of how long you live, trumping whether you smoke or are obese." A major study of 10,000 American men aged twenty to eighty-two confirmed that, over the course of five years, those who were the least aerobically fit were the most likely to die of all causes and at all ages. Conversely, the fifth that were the most fit were the least likely to die of any cause.

But this encouraging bit of news (or discouraging, if you sat in a chair all day) did not answer a more practical question: just how much running (or other aerobic activity) was enough? Even those committed to keeping up on the research could be excused for their bewilderment. Every year a new study produced a new set of guidelines and new recommendations, much of it contradictory. Some studies stressed duration as most beneficial, some high-intensity interval sprints. A recent study at the Cooper Institute found that the *speed* with which a middle-aged man or woman ran a mile predicted the risk of heart disease decades later. It seemed to put in bold at least one shared belief: the more exercise, the better.

But even that consensus had its detractors. Prominent among them was Steven Blair, one of Cooper's own scientists who had served as director of research at the institute. A marathoner himself, he was a firm believer that the best exercise was vigorous exercise. In 1989, however, he turned apostate when the *Journal of the American Medical Association* published the results of his study of 13,000 adults who had come to the institute to have their physical fitness assessed. The study then tracked their health for eight years, and no one was more surprised at the results than Blair. The greatest gains came from those who exercised only modestly, enough to climb from the lowest quintile, those who were virtually sedentary, into the next quintile up. The Blair study had its limits: demographics (almost all participants were white professionals), self-selection (motivated to improve their health), and lack of control group (Blair thought it unethical to require half the participants to do nothing). But the message was clear: "Moderate levels of physical fitness that are attainable by most adults," concluded the study, "appear to be protective against early mortality."

Other research confirmed these results. A major study at Harvard Medical School tracked almost 75,000 middle-aged female nurses and, in 1999, reported that walking three or four hours a week significantly reduced the risk of heart disease. More vigorous exercise made no difference. The implications were enormous for those most at risk, those who stayed sedentary because they *were* at risk, and would be frightened off with visions of a marathon or a high-intensity Spinning class. "A lot of [those] people would be so daunted that they wouldn't even try," said Michael Lauer, a cardiologist and research director at the Cleveland Clinic. "My parents always wanted me to be above average, but this is one area where average is fine."

The moderate-is-fine camp got another boost in June 2012 at the annual meeting of the American College of Sports Medicine. In her *Times* phys-ed column, Reynolds announced "the newest and perhaps most compelling of the studies" in which researchers had combed the health records of 52,656 American adults who had undergone physicals at the Cooper Institute between 1971 and 2002, checking death rates against running activity. Those who ran one to twenty miles a week at an average pace of ten or eleven minutes a mile—basically jogging—outlived the nonrunners, not surprisingly, but also, *very* surprisingly, those who ran faster and longer. "More running is not needed to produce extra health and mortality benefits," said Dr. Carl J. Lavie, medical director of cardiac rehabilitation and prevention at the Ochsner Medical Center in New Orleans and the study's author. "If anything, it appears that less running is associated with the best protection from mortality risk. More is not better, and actually, more could be worse."

A kind of uneasy consensus emerged from all this research and all these studies. A sensible standard of exercise was 150 minutes a week of moderate activity, such as five 30-minute walks. Doing much more was likely beneficial, but it would not significantly raise the benefits. Yet—and the subject of fitness always comes with a *yet*—surely the conversation should not begin and end with aerobic fitness. True, modest exercise such as jogging could increase a person's life span, but what about strength and flexibility? Weren't these also key components of a healthy body?

Of course they were. For young people, building muscle was important if they participated in sports and wanted to improve performance and lessen the risk of injury. For anyone, hefting a roll-on suitcase into an airplane's overhead bin was a test of upper-body strength. Strength became more critical in later years; as the body aged it lost muscle mass, and bone density dropped. Brittle bones could turn common tumbles into life-threatening events.

Flexibility, too, became more critical to fitness with age. Shorter, tightened muscles led to strains and rupture. A sense of balance reduced the risk of serious falls. (It is why both yoga and Pilates, though largely anaerobic, can be of such use to older people.) As with so many areas in fitness, however, there was continuing dispute as to what was useful exercise and what was wasted effort. For the casual consumer, the blizzard of advice could be overwhelming. Hundreds of books and DVDs promoted ever more effective exercise, while dozens of magazines competed with new schemes and "secret" star workouts — even as a small cadre of "experts" plumbed the research for hard data.

Even dismissing the cruder cover-line appeals to vanity — "monster muscles" and "rock-hard abs" — there is still plenty of room for dissension. Stretching, for instance, has long been a commonplace tenet among coaches and personal trainers. But recent research suggests its value may be greatly exaggerated — or worse. A study of college-age competitive runners at Florida State University in Tallahassee found that preparing for an hour's treadmill run with a sixteen-minute stretch routine — instead of just sitting around quietly — *reduced* the runners' performance; they covered less distance and consumed more oxygen and calories doing so. "Static stretching should be avoided before endurance events," concluded the scientists.

A much larger study followed 1,400 recreational runners over a three-month period; half stretched and half did not. A predictable number suffered minor injuries that caused them to miss training days — but there was no difference between the stretchers and the nonstretchers.

These and other studies were scrutinized by Reynolds in her book *The First 20 Minutes*. In it she acknowledged the value of "dynamic stretching" — working the specific muscles that were about to be employed in a sport or activity — but devoted much more space to exploding another myth: the value of warm-ups. In general, wrote Reynolds, warm-ups were more likely to tire athletes than help them improve performance and concluded this section, "Stretching the Truth," with a researcher's comment: "Less is more." She was joined in this assessment by *Times* colleague Gina Kolata, who quoted a different researcher in her book *Ultimate Fitness* who said, "There were experiments in which people did exercise with or without stretching and it didn't seem to make any difference."

Reynolds pounced on another "given" in her book: a strong core. It was long assumed that the firmer the midsection, the better the athlete.

Not so, she wrote. A study of NCAA Division I football players at the powerhouse Indiana University tested core-section strength and then measured their performance in dashes, leaps, and other challenges. In general, the players with the most rock-solid cores were no better at the sports-specific tests than those with feebler middles. The results astonished Dr. Thomas Nesser, a professor of physical education at Indiana who had conducted the study. "'I can't tell you how many times I ran the numbers and checked and re-checked the results,' he says. 'I couldn't believe it.'"

A study with nonathlete collegians confirmed the findings. There was little correlation between robust core muscles and athleticism. Another study of collegiate rowers found that after eight weeks of an arduous core-exercise regimen — on top of their normal workout — the rowers had great-looking abs but performed no better in a rowing-machine time trial. Nesser announced that the study pointed to the need to focus on "functional fitness" — building up the body in areas where it is weak, developing enough strength to make our bodies function better — "in sport and in life," added the helpful Reynolds.

Look hard enough and there were studies to confirm that most any workout — strengthening the core, becoming elastic enough to rest your elbows on the floor — might yield less than useful results. That said, few were prepared for the megastudy that came out mid-2012, reporting that some exercise could actually *increase* risks to the heart. Examining six other studies involving 1,687 people, the published paper found that 10 percent of the participants actually got worse on at least one of the measures related to heart disease.

This startling news, which made the front page of the *New York Times*, came from researchers with impressive bona fides and was endorsed by a top expert in the field, Dr. Michael Lauer, director of the Division of Cardiovascular Sciences at the National Heart, Lung, and Blood Institute, the lead federal research institute on heart disease and strokes. "It is an interesting and well-done study," said Lauer.

There were predictable howls of dismay. "There are a lot of people out there looking for any excuse not to exercise," lamented one expert. "This might be an excuse for them to say, 'Oh, I must be one of those ten percent.'"

And yet — yet! — it would be wrong to dismiss the tangible result of so much effort. There is, after all, great benefit to be had from exercise — much of it affecting the brain as much as the body. Jake Steinfeld was only one in a long line of gym rats when he exclaimed, "I just *love* working out!" The stars of *Pumping Iron* were mostly a merry band, the contorted agony of their training faces merely the price of more lasting pleasure. Some of that good cheer was satisfaction, the pride of accomplishment and sense of achievement (or relief) that awaited the end of any workout. But extreme effort brought with it other rewards: the flush of exhilaration Jim Fixx felt at the end of his daily run, often characterized as the "runner's high" and more specifically laid to the flood of morphine-like chemicals that could induce a kind of euphoria.

The notion of an "endorphin rush" is both a commonplace and a mystery. There is endless research that attempts to locate a particular brain chemical or group of endorphins that get activated during exercise. For compulsive exercisers, they may resemble a drug addict's "fix" — their absence triggering a mild form of morphine withdrawal. Kolata is wary of mythologizing the role of these natural opiates, though she is quick to offer anecdotal evidence that, once you start to exercise, there is no denying the addictive allure. Describing a two-day work stint in which she could not get to the gym, she became tired, "dragged down by the intense effort and pressure of the job." She finally seized a two-hour window of opportunity. "I dashed to Gold's Gym in time for the 7:00 p.m. Spinning class. I pushed myself hard and by the time it was over, I felt renewed, totally invigorated, euphoric. I knew, once again, why I love exercise."

There will, of course, always be those who take up exercise for another reason entirely: simply to look good. The history of fitness has long been propelled by the presumed benefits of appearance, and that motive served many well. Untold thousands of comic-book readers owed their new confidence to the programs they purchased from Charles Atlas. Fonda inspired an entire generation of women to exercise, many because they hoped to look as good as she did. The problem comes when the image of fitness trumps its substance. We may be smart enough now to dismiss the grotesque bulging biceps on the covers of muscle fan books, but what about the six-pack abs that are commonly used to sell high-priced underwear and designer jeans? What about the ripped torsos that adorn the covers of *Men's Health*, the presumptive bible of, well, men's health? A washboard stomach may reflect well in the mirror but, in truth, offers little if no actual health benefit. Men's obsession with "Ab Flab" and the urge to present a rigid, iron-hard middle may well be rooted in psychological issues and the need to retain control in a world that is increasingly threatened by "softer" women. Even that mantra of many personal trainers—"Draw your stomach into your navel"—has been cited by some exercise experts as counterproductive and possibly harmful to the spine if done during the wrong phase of a workout. Of course fit-focused women's magazines—the likes of *Shape* and *Self*, with their covers of impossibly taut tummies—are no less at fault for confusing a sexual trigger with evidence of true well-being.

It is in the nature of our merchandising culture to sell aspiration, but that habit is not helpful when it comes to fostering a fuller, more informed notion of fitness. It is not helpful when we marginalize a great sector of the population, those who would benefit most from exercise, because they do not conform to the body types whom club owners flaunt on their sexy billboards and promotional videos.

THE SHAPE OF THE FUTURE

"Exercise needs to become a cultural priority," says Richard Cotton, president of the ACSM, "and in some respects it is. There's so much in the public space about the value of physical activity and eating well as it relates to quality of life. The problem is we end up preaching to the choir."

It is, to be sure, a very large choir. If one requirement of an exercise habit is access to facilities, there is no shortage of churches. There are fitness facilities everywhere, ranging from branded multisport clubs to mom-and-pop studios. More and more companies offer onsite gyms; even modest hotels have workout rooms. There are yoga studios in airports and Pilates classes at YMCAs. Personal trainers make home visits, and not all will bankrupt the budget. A discerning consumer can do plenty with home equipment or DVDs. With all these options, there are fewer and fewer excuses to stay planted on the living-room sofa. The challenge is getting started. The challenge is motivation.

The pursuit of fitness has undergone vast changes in America over the past century. Its earliest evangelists, the likes of Macfadden, roused a rabid following to enshrine the body and what was put into it. Atlas recruited the common man to the cause. The buff culture spread from the sands of Muscle Beach to the big-screen stars of Hollywood and millions of fans. Equipment breakthroughs made exercise easier and more effective. Spurred by Cooper, the country embraced aerobics and the value of cardiovascular exercise, and America hit the jogging path. Women, inspired by the likes of Fonda and the dance divas, took the lead in group exercise. In the eighties the launch of the health club boom heralded a new era in which all that fitness enthusiasts had promoted became suddenly available in one place and with social benefits. Clubs became so widespread and popular that Phillip Mills did not exaggerate when he called them the arena of "the world's biggest adult sport, bigger than soccer, golf, and tennis combined."

Yet ultimately growth stagnated; club membership stalled at 15 percent, and Mills thinks he knows why. "Our industry hasn't seen a lot of innovation in the last five years," he says. "Clubs have become a boring sport." For all their reach, for all their transformative influence, Mills believes, clubs have failed to make good on their promise. He views the popularity of "budget" clubs, the ones that charge ten dollars, as evidence that members have lost faith in what a true health club should provide. He detailed those ideas in a 2010 "Future of Fitness" white paper he sponsored that argued for new priorities. Citing the "fragmentation" of society — the loss of meaningful places for social interaction — he urged that clubs play more of a community role. Not surprisingly, he touted group exercise as a promising area. So was small group training. So were "clubs within a club" — like-minded members who cooked, wine-tasted, read books, attended nutrition lectures, or group-trained for races or charity cycle rides. "No one ever left a gym because they made too many friends," said Mills.

He urged a design facelift. "If we tried very hard to create the worst possible environment for exercise," he said, "we would come up with something much like the modern group exercise room. With its wall-to-wall mirrors, white color scheme and bright lighting, it's a cold intimidating space that induces self-consciousness. It's more like a hospital operating room than a place where you would hang out for fun."

Finally, perhaps most critically, Mills urged that clubs play a more educational role for their members, helping to remedy the poor nutrition and harmful habits of a sedentary culture, a situation he detailed in his book *Globesity*. "True 'health' clubs will exist only when we help people grow from interested party to hobbyist to expert to fanatic when it comes to both their own health and the well-being of their wider community. Quite simply," said Mills, "we need to become health educators."

One challenge Mills and others face is the habit of denial. Americans may be quick to register alarming data—but often believe the risk belongs to others, not themselves. In a National Cancer Awareness Survey, 70 percent of those polled said they believed that healthy living could reduce the risk of cancer, but less than 30 percent attributed their personal cancer risk to unhealthy behaviors such as poor nutrition, lack of exercise, or weight gain. Another survey, this from Destiny Health, found that two-thirds of Americans saw themselves as "physically active," and only 30 percent believed they were overweight. "The harsh reality," said Destiny's chief medical officer, Dr. Charles Schutz, "is that the Department of Health and Human Services literally reverses those numbers." The Destiny study was reported with this headline: "American Idle Is Killing Us: Unhealthy Optimism about Health Weighing Americans Down."

The fitness industry, at least some of it, is making attempts to narrow this "knowledge gap." Cotton, for one, is eager to promote a major initiative at the ACSM called "Exercise Is Medicine." It is aimed at recruiting the medical profession and borrows from what is known as the Kaiser System. Patients who come in for checkups with doctors routinely have their heart rate monitored, blood pressure checked, levels of serum cholesterol measured; in the Kaiser System, they are asked two additional questions: "How many times a week do you exercise?" and "How many minutes per session?" The doctor then feeds the answers into a computer program. If the numbers do not multiply to 150 minutes—the federal guideline for acceptable exercise—the computer screen goes red.

Getting started is one priority. Turning an experiment into a habit is often trickier. People with the best of intentions may give gym membership a whirl or hire a personal trainer and then just as quickly quit. Cotton, whose group certifies trainers, lays some of the blame on exercise professionals. "For too long, trainers have been working in the mode of body technicians rather than behavioral change agents. They put together great programs and worked all the muscles, but they didn't do anything with what's going on between a client's ears."

If that strategy changes, it will owe much to a model called "Stages of Change" (SOC) originally developed at the University of Rhode Island in the late 1970s and early 1980s as a means to help smokers give up their habit. It has since been applied to a broad range of behaviors that include weight loss, injury prevention, and overcoming alcohol and drug problems. The idea is that people go through stages on their way to successful change. Somewhat analogous to the stages of grief, it requires each individual to fully embrace each stage before moving on; the stages cannot be hurried or imposed externally. The ACSM is in the process of incorporating the SOC model into its certification exam for trainers, and Cotton believes it will "add depth to the profession" and greatly support people in "sustainable behavior change."

Change cannot come too soon. In addition to the alarm about obesity and its attendant ills, there is concern that America's youth are increasingly at risk. Fewer and fewer children walk to school, a key to physical activity. In budget-conscious times and with schools pressed to put up high academic numbers, gym class is often first to suffer a cutback. Teens and preteens often pass up athletics and exercise in favor of addictive onscreen options or, competing to get into schools or land jobs, are overscheduled by anxious parents and are simply too busy.

Fortunately, all is not gloom and doom. The benefits of exercise have never been more zealously promoted. More and more, physicians are telling their patients they need to get up and out and move. Books and magazines flood the market with sane workout options; columnists like the *Times*'s Reynolds provide constant new information. The blizzard of studies and research may leave some readers scratching their heads, but the good news is: increasing numbers of experts are studying exercise to maximize its benefits for young and old. Running has never been more popular. Group fitness is enjoying a boom—and so are hard-core boot camps and triathlons. The popularity of yoga and Pilates has yet to show signs of peaking. Health clubs, the most visible face of fitness, are a vital source of exciting new workout ideas. Businesses are promoting fitness, if largely out of self-interest. In its booklet *The Economic Benefits of Regular Exercise*, IHRSA cites the major savings in health care costs that employers reap from workers who are fit. In Washington IHRSA's lobbying efforts were key in reintroducing the Workforce Health Improvement Program, which would reclassify employer-provided fitness memberships as nontaxable income. IHRSA also pressed Congress to pass the PHIT, or Personal Health Investment Today, Act, which would allow employers to pay for gym memberships.

There is no simple solution to combating obesity or the threat of inertial America, but singly and together these developments offer hope that a fitter future awaits. If so, we owe a debt to the men and women who came before — the muscle heads and joggers, the nutritional zealots and barbell salesmen, the machine inventors and aerobics divas. The day of the great pioneers may have come to a close, but what they worked for so passionately endures. It is the promise that we can all live longer, richer lives if we learn to attend to our bodies.

Notes

1. THE SHAPE OF HISTORY

3 **"We Are Weak":** Jan Todd, "The Classical Ideal and Its Impact on the Search for Suitable Exercise: 1774–1830," *Iron Game History* 2, no. 4 (1992): 7.

3 **Mortified by Napoleon's defeat:** Michael Anton Budd, *The Sculpture Machine: Physical Culture and Body Politics in the Age of Empire* (New York: New York University Press, 1997), 16.

3 **Most remarkably, he filled it:** Stephen Tharrett, Frank O'Rourke, and James A. Peterson, *Legends of Fitness* (Monterey CA: Healthy Learning, 2011), 145.

3 **His fanatic anti-Semitism:** Claire E. Nolte, "The German Turnverein," in *Encyclopedia of the 1848 Revolutions* (2005), edited by James Chastain, http://www.ohio.edu/chastain/.

3 **His biography would have been fantastic:** David L. Chapman, "Hippolyte Triat," *Iron Game History* 4, no. 1 (1995): 3.

4 **The less privileged could buy shares:** Tharrett, O'Rourke, and Peterson, *Legends of Fitness*, 27.

4 **In 1848, riding the wave:** Tharrett, O'Rourke, and Peterson, *Legends of Fitness*, 29.

4 **"[It is] a good thing":** Quoted in Tony Ladd and James A. Mathisen, *Muscular Christianity: Evangelical Protestants and the Development of American Sport* (Peabody MA: BridgePoint Books, 1999), 13–14.

5 **A Frenchman and rabid Anglophile:** Frank Deford, "Britannia Rules the Games," *Sports Illustrated*, July–August 2012, 42–44.

5 **"Games conduce not merely to physical":** Quoted in Ladd and Mathisen, *Muscular Christianity*, 106.

5 **"Bodily vigor is a moral agent":** James C. Whorton, *Crusaders for Fitness* (Princeton NJ: Princeton University Press, 1982), 290.

5 **There was added urgency:** Harvey Green, *Fit for America: Health, Fitness, Sport in American Society* (Baltimore: Johns Hopkins University Press, 1986), 215.

6 **"Muscular posing's conflation":** Budd, *Sculpture Machine*, 75.

6 **Weston the Pedestrian:** Green, *Fit for America*, 205.

8 **"In his assertion that thorough mastication":** Green, *Fit for America*, 299.

8 **"I Fletcherize, and that's my life":** Green, *Fit for America*, 297.

8 **The verb *Fletcherize*:** Green, *Fit for America*, 295.

2. SELLING THE BODY BEAUTIFUL, 1900–1930S

11 **"You were no one":** Josh Buck, "Sandow: No Folly with Ziegfeld's First Glorification," *Iron Game History* 5, no. 1 (1998): 30.

12 **Attila was so impressed:** David L. Chapman, "Sandow's First Triumph," *Iron Game History* 3, no. 3 (1994): 3.

12 **"running your hand over corrugated iron":** David L. Chapman, *Sandow the Magnificent* (Urbana: University of Illinois Press, 1994), 46.

13 **The man who entered:** Buck, "Sandow," 29.

13 **Ziegfeld, his star's irrepressible keeper:** Chapman, *Sandow the Magnificent*, 91.

14 **As pointed out by one Joyce scholar:** Brandon R. Kerschner, "The World's Strongest Man: Joyce or Sandow?," *James Joyce Quarterly* 30, no. 4 (1993): 667–93, cited in Martina Vike, "A Feat of Strength in 'Ithaca': Eugen Sandow and Physical Culture in Joyce's *Ulysses*," *Journal of Modern Literature* (Indiana University Press) (Fall 2006): 129–39.

14 **Sandow was the obvious model:** Chapman, *Sandow the Magnificent*, 150.

14 **He had a serious admirer:** Harold Weiss, "Sherlock Holmes, Arthur Conan Doyle, and the 'Iron Pills,'" *Iron Game History* (March 1991): 21.

15 **News reports had him dying:** Chapman, *Sandow the Magnificent*, 184–86.

15 **The magnificent plaster cast:** Chapman, *Sandow the Magnificent*, 139.

16 **Macfadden had grown up dirt-poor:** Much biographical information owed to Mark Adams, *Mr. America: How Muscular Millionaire Bernarr Macfadden Transformed the Nation through Sex, Salad, and the Ultimate Starvation Diet* (New York: HarperCollins, 2009).

17 **between 1830 and 1890:** Adams, *Mr. America*, 43.

17 **"He freely used celebrities":** Adams, *Mr. America*, 44.

17 **Reputing Victorian notions of female frailty:** Jan Todd, "Bernarr Macfadden: Reformer of Feminine Form," *Iron Game History* 1, nos. 4–5 (1991): 5–6.

18 **At its peak Macfadden's publishing empire:** Ben Yagoda, "The True Story of Bernarr Macfadden," *American Heritage* 33, no. 1 (1981): 26.

18 **The *Graphic* was also where:** Adams, *Mr. America*, 135–37.

18 **True believers included novelist Upton Sinclair:** Adams, *Mr. America*, 73.

19 **Some of his practices were worse:** Yagoda, "The True Story of Bernarr Macfadden," 90.

19 **Who but Macfadden would have tapped:** Yagoda, "The True Story of Bernarr Macfadden," 170.

20 **Mary penned a torrid:** Yagoda, "The True Story of Bernarr Macfadden," 4.

21 **Charles Atlas was born:** Much biographical information derived from Charles Gaines, *Yours in Perfect Manhood: Charles Atlas* (New York: Simon and Schuster, 1982).

22 **Perhaps it was "merely remarkable coincidence":** Adams, *Mr. America*, 113–14.

22 **It was saved by a twenty-one-year-old:** Gaines, *Yours in Perfect Manhood*, 65.

24 **"Get up immediately on awakening":** Documents from the Charles Atlas Collection in the Smithsonian Museum, Washington DC.

24 **"What's the matter with those fellows":** Gaines, *Yours in Perfect Manhood*, 82.

24 **"Live clean, think clean":** Gaines, *Yours in Perfect Manhood*, 92.

25 **Joe Weider, the Canadian bodybuilder:** Joe Weider, e-mail to the author, September 8, 2008.

25 **"Charles Atlas built his body":** Bill Pearl, *Legends of the Iron Game* (Phoenix OR: Bill Pearl Enterprises, 2010), 1:202.

26 **He had grown up:** Much biographical information owed to John D. Fair, *Muscletown USA: Bob Hoffman and the Manly Culture of York Barbell* (University Park: Pennsylvania State University Press, 1999).

27 **"The only thing she faults me for":** Terry Todd, "Remembering Bob Hoffman," *Iron Game History* 3, no. 1 (1993): 20.

27 **Amused by his "Jovean ability":** T. Todd, "Remembering Bob Hoffman," 23.

27 **He was a major late-life philanthropist:** T. Todd, "Remembering Bob Hoffman," 23.

27 **Hoffman mixing an unpalatable brew:** Jim Murray, "More Memories of Bob Hoffman," *Iron Game History* 3, no. 2 (1994): 6.

28 **Ziegler was a colorful character:** Fair, *Muscletown USA*, 158.

28 **Luring his counterpart:** Justin Peters, "The Doctor Who Brought Steroids to America," *Slate*, February 18, 2005, 1.

28 **CIBA unleashed a drug:** Peters, "Steroids to America," 1.

29 **"I wish I'd never heard":** Pearl, *Legends of the Iron Game*, 1:234.

29 **The Internal Revenue Service:** Fair, *Muscletown USA*, 175.

29 **charged him with "fixing" physique contests:** Fair, *Muscletown USA*, 177.

29 **"A boobybuilder":** Fair, *Muscletown USA*, 169.

30 **"I was able to withstand":** T. Todd, "Remembering Bob Hoffman," 2.

3. AMERICA SHAPES UP, 1930S–1950S

32 **There was Paula Unger Boelsems:** Marla Matzer Rose, *Muscle Beach: Where the Best Bodies in the World Started a Fitness Revolution* (New York: LA Weekly Books/St. Martin's Press, 2001), 40–45.

32 **"At the end of the depression":** Jan Todd, "The Legacy of Pudgy Stockton," *Iron Game History* 2, no. 1 (1992): 5.

32 **Trimmed down, she finally:** Rose, *Muscle Beach*, 49.

33 **By the end of the 1940s:** J. Todd, "Legacy of Pudgy Stockton," 6.

33 **Known as "Genial George":** Pearl, *Legends of the Iron Game*, 3:129.

33 **His own star turn:** Rose, *Muscle Beach*, 82.

34 **"You'd know him a mile away":** Joe Weider and Ben Weider, *Brothers of Iron* (Champaign IL: Sports Publishing, 2006), 92.

34 **refusing to believe that "Italians could make a western":** John Francis Lane, "Steve Reeves: Putting Muscle and Myth in the Movies," *Guardian*, May 5, 2000.

35 **The highlight had West lounging:** Rose, *Muscle Beach* (citing recollection of Armand Tanny), 77.

36 **"Two long steep staircases":** Randy Roach, *Muscle, Smoke, and Mirrors* (Bloomington IN: AuthorHouse, 2008), 1:375.

38 **"Entering a Tanny Health Center":** "Vic Tanny: America's Greatest Health Educator," *Wisdom* (Wisdom Society), December 1961.

38 **His extravagance knew no bounds:** Josh Buick, "The Evolution of Health Clubs," *Club Industry* (December 1, 1999).

38 **"Volume is what counts":** Tharrett, O'Rourke, and Peterson, *Legends of Fitness*, 69.

39 **There were so many complaints:** Tharrett, O'Rourke, and Peterson, *Legends of Fitness*, 69–70.

39 **maintained a strict raw-food diet:** Roach, *Muscle, Smoke, and Mirrors*, 1:182–83.

39 **"Rumors may have reached you":** Roach, *Muscle, Smoke, and Mirrors*, 1:372.

40 **"At 15 I knew":** Huston Horn, "LaLanne: A Treat and a Treatment," *Sports Illustrated*, December 19, 1960. See also Roach, *Muscle, Smoke, and Mirrors*, 1:110.

40 **Armand Tanny recalled visiting:** Roach, *Muscle, Smoke, and Mirrors*, 1:112.

41 **"You know, students":** Video from http://www.JackLaLanne.com.

41 **In Los Angeles:** Horn, "LaLanne."

42 **"remarkable mix of wheat germ":** "Helpmate for Herenow," *Newsweek*, July 25, 1960, 102.

42 **"What LaLanne was selling":** Bob Ottum, "Look, Mom, I'm an Institution," *Sports Illustrated*, November 23, 1981.

42 **"wherever the family of man":** Horn, "LaLanne."

42 **"Man, she has a terrific body":** "Helpmate for Herenow."

43 **His most celebrated stunt:** Pearl, *Legends of the Iron Game*, 1:321.

44 **The evidence had first appeared:** History of the President's Council on Physical Fitness and Sports (1956–2006), http://www.fitness.gov/about/history.

44 **"the greatest array of U.S. sports stars":** Robert H. Boyle, "The Report That Shocked the President," *Sports Illustrated*, August 15, 1955.

44 **The woman had put up a record:** "Bonnie Prudden: A Gunks Pioneer," *Climberism*, January 18, 2012.

44 **As a four-year-old:** Bonnie Prudden, unpublished autobiography, courtesy of Myotherapy, Tucson AZ.

45 **"I was horrified":** Prudden, unpublished autobiography.

46 **Walter Lippmann claimed that America:** Marc Richards, "The Cold War's 'Soft Recruits,'" *Peace Review* (September 1998).

47 **"In a very real and immediate sense":** President-Elect John F. Kennedy, "The Soft American," *Sports Illustrated*, December 26, 1960.

47 **the following year she appeared:** *Sports Illustrated*, August 5, 1957.

47 **"Leotards and tights were signals to exercise":** Prudden, unpublished autobiography.

4. THE MACHINE AGE, 1960S–1970S

50 **It was 1974 when Wilson:** Ray Wilson, phone interview with the author, May 2012.

51 **"Arthur was a genius":** Wilson, interview.

52 **"Aerobic exercises":** Kirk Semple, "The Rise of the Machines," *New York Times*, September 2, 2007.

52 **"Arthur could be downright dangerous":** Quoted in Roach, *Muscle, Smoke, and Mirrors*, 2:313; see also 558.

53 **He was even questioned:** Roach, *Muscle, Smoke, and Mirrors*, 2:322.

54 **"He was a very, *very* intense person":** Gary Jones, phone interview with the author, December 2011.

54 **When Gary got home:** Jones, interview.

55 **"There are also machines":** Charles Gaines and George Butler, *Pumping Iron: The Art and Sport of Bodybuilding.*

55 **"Sales of his units":** Roach, *Muscle, Smoke, and Mirrors*, 2:347.

55 **"He understood what I wanted to do":** Ellington Darden, phone interview with the author, August 2012.

56 **"A gun is like a tourniquet":** Video of *Late Night with David Letterman*, August 12, 1982.

56 **He was not happy:** Jones, interview.

57 **"Arthur taught me a lot":** Jones, interview.

57 **He had grown up dirt-poor:** Wilson, interview.

58 **"The spa," Wilson admitted:** E-mail posted to friends on the occasion of Delmonteque's death in 2012.

58 **"When the weights came":** Autobiography from his website, http://www.bobdelmonteque.com.

58 **"We both went kind of bananas":** Wilson, interview.

60 **"Here's the deal":** Wilson, interview.

61 **Thus began a saga:** Wilson, interview.

61 **Nieto had suffered miserably:** Augie Nieto, interview with the author, Corona del Mar, California, December 2006.

62 **"I knew that exercise":** Nieto, interview.

63 **By the late 1970s:** Tharrett, O'Rourke, and Peterson, *Legends of Fitness*, 148.

63 **"It was," said Nieto:** Nieto, interview.

63 **In 1997 Nieto sold the company again:** Chris Clawson, CEO of Life Time Fitness, interview with the author, Schiller Park, Illinois, February 2012.

66 **One of the more dogged:** Siri Galliano, phone interview with the author, January 2012.

66 **Pilates then was already married:** Stacey Redfield-Dreisbach, "Chasing Joe Pilates," unpublished manuscript.

67 **"Contrology is a complete coordination":** Joseph Pilates, *Return to Life through Contrology*, originally published in 1945, reprinted in 1998 by Presentation Dynamics of Ashland, Oregon.

68 **Every summer he and Clara:** Video courtesy of Mary Bowen.

68 **"There was a fire":** Mary Bowen, interview with the author, New York City, February 2012.

5. GOTTA MOVE, 1960S–1980S

71 **"The sophisticated life":** Gina Kolata, *Ultimate Fitness* (New York: Farrar, Straus, and Giroux, 2003), 44.

72 **"I thought I was having a heart attack":** Ken Cooper, phone interview with the author, February 2012.

73 **Cooper liked to tell the tale:** Amy George, "Aerobics: 40 Years of Changing Lives," *Cooperhealth*, Fall 2008.

74 **"Doctor, I don't care":** Kenneth H. Cooper, *Aerobics* (New York: M. Evans, in association with Lippincott, 1968), 82.

76 **He made headlines again:** John Brant, "Frank's Story," *Runner's World*, August 31, 2011.

76 **"'Why does your father'":** Andrew Sheehan, *Chasing the Hawk: Looking for My Father, Finding Myself* (New York: Delacorte Press, 2001), quoted in Kolata, *Ultimate Fitness*, 46.

76 **"Being a doctor's not a big deal":** Jonathan Black, "What Makes George Run?," *Runner* (May 1981): 26.

77 **"Frank Shorter invented running":** James Fixx, *Jackpot!* (New York: Random House, 1982), 115.

77 **The magazine *Runner's World*:** Jack W. Berryman, *Out of Many, One: A History of the American College of Sports Medicine* (Champaign IL: Human Kinetics, 1995), 146.

78 **"I noticed some surprising psychological benefits":** Quoted in Kolata, *Ultimate Fitness*, 47.

79 **"best and quickest way":** Cooper, *Aerobics*, 138.

80 **When Neil was assigned:** Details here and following are from Beth Swanson, "The Rise of Aerobic Dance" (master's thesis, University of California, San Diego, 1994).

81 **In 1981 her company:** Swanson, "Rise of Aerobic Dance," 167.

81 **Jazzercise instructors were making:** Swanson, "Rise of Aerobic Dance," 189.

82 **A woman named Martha Rounds:** Swanson, "Rise of Aerobic Dance."

83 **The high point:** Patricia Bosworth, *Jane Fonda: The Private Life of a Public Woman* (Boston and New York: Houghton Mifflin Harcourt, 2011), 456.

84 **"You know what I should have said":** *New Yorker*, May 9, 2011, 58.

85 **Brainstorming, she had even considered:** Bosworth, *Jane Fonda*.

85 **"You could open a studio":** Bosworth, *Jane Fonda*, 480.

85 **dispatched her spy to Century City:** Bosworth, *Jane Fonda*, 438.

85 **"Jane helped me":** Bosworth, *Jane Fonda*, 480.

85 **He agreed but, knowing nothing about aerobics:** *Chicago Tribune*, July 4, 2012, "Business," 3.

86 **"I didn't know what a video *was*":** Fonda accepting the Jack LaLanne Award at the 2012 IDEA convention.

86 **training the state's future governor:** Jill Ross, founder and president of Collage Video, phone interview with the author, August 2012.

86 **"Jane Fonda, Raquel Welch":** Kathy Larkin, syndicated newspapers, December 4, 1983.

86 **"I've always had a hyper kind of energy":** Larkin, syndicated newspapers.

87 **"Though I waddle through the valley":** Kathy MacKay, "Richard Simmons, the Sultan of Svelte, Applies Both the Carrot and the Schtick," *People*, November 2, 1981, 95.

88 **"monster of the morning":** MacKay, "Richard Simmons."

88 **Though he never discussed:** Kevin Pang, "The Many Secrets of Richard Simmons," *Chicago Tribune*, June 4, 2008.

88 **"blend of queer sensibility":** Rhonda Garelick, "Outrageous Dieting: The Camp Performance of Richard Simmons," *Postmodern Culture* (Oxford University Press) 6, no. 1 (1995).

88 **tooled around Beverly Hills:** MacKay, "Richard Simmons."

88 **The year he turned sixty:** Pang, "Many Secrets," 1.

90 **his college classmates pigeonholed him:** Kateri Drexler, *Icons of Business: An Encyclopedia of Mavericks, Movers, and Shakers* (Westport CT: Greenwood, 2007), 2:271.

90 **"Those who had liked":** J. B. Strasser and Laurie Becklund, *Swoosh: The Story of Nike and the Men Who Played There* (New York: Harcourt, Brace, Jovanovich, 1991), 11.

91 **The "Swoosh" logo was provided:** Strasser and Becklund, *Swoosh*, 126.
91 **He had been drinking:** Strasser and Becklund, *Swoosh*, 505.
92 **In fact, the design:** Phil Trotter, phone interview with the author, July 2012.
92 **selling more than $100 million:** Strasser and Becklund, *Swoosh*, 574.
92 **the well-known miler Marty Liquori:** "Athletic Shoe Boom Slows to a Fast Walk," *Chicago Tribune*, March 8, 1987.
92 **Fireman was more cautious:** "Athletic Shoe Boom."
93 **"it seemed the thing":** Gin Miller, phone interview with the author, July 2012.
94 **She partnered with the owners:** Trotter, interview.
94 **"That's what protected me":** Miller, interview.
94 **Reebok had a ready-made test group:** Miller, interview.
95 **"What makes fitness great?":** Miller, interview.

6. THE BUFF CULTURE, 1970S–1990S

98 **"I was frightened of being ignorant":** Weider and Weider, *Brothers of Iron*, 12.
99 **"They became an embarrassment I didn't need":** Weider and Weider, *Brothers of Iron*, 115.
99 **"the longest craziest pissing match":** Weider and Weider, *Brothers of Iron*, 99.
99 **"Hoffman once called me a kike":** Weider and Weider, *Brothers of Iron*, 99.
100 **"there was no clinic as such":** Roach, *Muscle, Smoke, and Mirrors*, 1:234.
101 **"Give me a break!":** Weider and Weider, *Brothers of Iron*, 88.
101 **The showdown never happened:** Roach, *Muscle, Smoke, and Mirrors*, 1:154–55.
101 **"That guy," Weider would write:** Weider and Weider, *Brothers of Iron*, 89.
102 **"He probably felt a sense of nostalgia":** John D. Fair, "Hercules Meets Sealtest Dan," *Iron Game History* 6, no. 4 (2000): 33.
103 **"While Betty and Larry kicked around names":** Weider and Weider, *Brothers of Iron*, 158.
104 **"What he had in size":** Weider and Weider, *Brothers of Iron*, 163.
104 **"When the student is ready":** Weider and Weider, *Brothers of Iron*, 156.
105 **"Bodybuilding has advertised itself":** Gaines and Butler, *Pumping Iron*, introduction.
105 **"He caught her":** Gaines and Butler, *Pumping Iron*, 98.
106 **Several studies would find:** Bianca Hitt, "Reverse Anorexia in Bodybuilders," http://www.vanderbilt.edu/ans/psychology/health.
106 **"The '70s was the decade":** Bruce J. Schulman, *The Seventies* (Cambridge MA: Da Capo Press, 2002), 145.
108 **"The guys had nowhere to go":** Pearl, *Legends of the Iron Game*, 2:74.
108 **He never bought ads:** Paul Solotaroff, "Muscle Beach and the Dawn of Huge," *Men's Journal*, February 2012, 63.
108 **"If you got up":** Quoted in Laurence Leamer, *Fantastic: The Life of Arnold Schwarzenegger* (New York: St. Martin's Press, 2005), 58.

108 **He was born in the Austrian village:** Much biographical detail is owed to Leamer, *Fantastic.*

108 **"My hair was pulled":** Leamer, *Fantastic*, 15.

109 **Nor did he attend the funeral:** Leamer, *Fantastic*, 91–92.

110 **"He had contacted me":** Arnold Schwarzenegger and Douglas Kent Hall, *The Education of a Bodybuilder* (New York: Simon and Schuster, 1977), 94–95.

110 **Then they took the tapes:** Leamer, *Fantastic*, 59–60.

110 **"I found out right away":** Schwarzenegger and Kent, *Education of a Bodybuilder*, 95.

111 **"Nine-thirty, sharp":** Solotaroff, "Muscle Beach," 62.

111 **Most of the serious bodybuilders:** Solotaroff, "Muscle Beach," 62.

111 **Gold's was also the hub:** Solotaroff, "Muscle Beach," 64.

111 **"When a homosexual looks at a bodybuilder":** Gaines and Butler, *Pumping Iron*, 92.

113 **"Sure . . . and Ronald Reagan is going to be President":** Roach, *Muscle, Smoke, and Mirrors*, 2:96.

114 **"I couldn't have been a better pilot project":** Dan Isaacson, interview with the author, Los Angeles, March 2012.

114 **Mickey Rourke needed to look buff:** "Body Styler of the Rich and Famous," *Time*, December 2, 1985, 88.

115 **"I asked him, 'You sure that's okay?'":** Isaacson, interview.

115 **"It was hailing":** Jake Steinfeld, interview with the author, Los Angeles, March 2012.

116 **He met an actress:** Mary Fischer, "When Jake Steinfeld Barks, Spielberg, Presley, and Garr Jump (and Strech, and Bend)," *People*, May 9, 1983, 59.

116 **"It happened so fast":** Steinfeld, interview.

117 **"The only problem":** Fischer, "When Jake Steinfeld Barks," 59.

117 **Developed musculature was seen as "unsexing":** Maria Popova, review of *Venus with Biceps: A History of Muscular Women in Pictures*, by David L. Chapman and Patricia Vertinsky (Vancouver BC: Arsenal Pulp Press, 2010), *Atlantic*, November 24, 2011.

117 **When Macfadden staged a women's "physical culture contest":** Jan Todd and Desiree Harguess, "Doris Barrilleaux and the Beginnings of Modern Women's Bodybuilding," *Iron Game History* 11, no. 4 (2012): 10.

118 **"On to the fanny-swingers":** J. Todd and Harguess, "Doris Barrilleaux."

118 **In her book *Bodymakers* Leslie Heywood:** Leslie Heywood, *Bodymakers: A Cultural Anatomy of Women's Body Building* (New Brunswick NJ: Rutgers University Press, 1998).

118 **A second submission:** J. Todd and Harguess, "Doris Barrilleaux," 9.

119 **That credit goes to Henry McGhee:** J. Todd and Harguess, "Doris Barrilleaux," 19.

120 **"The gym is the world":** Heywood, *Bodymakers*, 3.

120 **"If you have an entirely new activity":** Jan Todd, interview with the author, Houston, Texas, July 2012.

120 **Heywood, for one, came to disdain:** Heywood, "Building Otherwise," in *Critical Readings in Bodybuilding* (New York: Routledge, 2012), 126.

120 **"[It] was enough to make me turn away":** Heywood, "Building Otherwise," 125.

7. PUMPING UP BUSINESS, 1980S–1990S

124 **Schwartz had captained his Yale tennis team:** Alan Schwartz, interview with the author, Chicago.

125 **The most ambitious opened:** Schwartz, interview.

126 **In the late 1960s:** Tharrett, O'Rourke, and Peterson, *Legends of Fitness*, 64.

126 **The blueprint for this transformation:** Tharrett, O'Rourke, and Peterson, *Legends of Fitness*, 154.

126 **Dibble, an industrial designer:** Obituary of Dale Dibble, *Club Insider* (February 19, 2012).

127 **Memberships soared:** Norm Cates, *Club Insider* (Clubinsider.com, December 17, 2010).

127 **"Traveling to his club, Cedardale":** Cates, *Club Insider*.

128 **Tinturi, a Finnish company:** Tharrett, O'Rourke, and Peterson, *Legends of Fitness*, 70.

129 **The "penetration rate":** Rick Caro, interview with the author, New York City, March 2012.

129 **The targeted marketing to senior executives:** Caro, interview.

130 **Fistfights landed him in juvenile court:** Susan Casey, "The World's Healthiest 75-Year-Old Man," *Esquire*, May 1, 2008.

130 **"When I got off the boat":** Casey, "World's Healthiest Man."

130 **"It was revolutionary":** Donahue Wildman, phone interview with the author, July 2012.

131 **When Ray Wilson opened:** Wildman, interview.

131 **"He just didn't have much faith":** Wildman, interview.

131 **A friend and next-door neighbor:** Wildman, interview.

132 **"I was always very ambitious":** Wildman, interview.

132 **Wildman's operation needed a fresh start:** Wildman, interview.

132 **"They made me an offer":** Wildman, interview.

133 **Its Holiday Health Clubs:** Pamela Kufahl, "Health Clubs of the 1990s," *Club Industry* (January 1, 2009).

133 **A college athlete and fitness enthusiast:** Mark Mastrov, interview with the author, San Ramon, California, November 2012.

134 **"He was an industry legend":** Mastrov, interview.

134 **"It was hand to mouth":** Mastrov, interview.

135 **"This is a very difficult industry":** Mastrov, interview.

135 **It was in this vacuum:** Tharrett, O'Rourke, and Peterson, *Legends of Fitness*, 92–93.

136 **The ACSM had been around:** Dick Cotton, phone interview with the author, July 2012.

136 **In 1975 the excitement of running:** http://www.acsm.org.

136 **When a respected Chicago gynecologist:** Berryman, *Out of Many, One*, 165–66.

137 **"Almost none of these teachers":** Kathie Davis, phone interview with the author, July 2012.

137 **For its first convention:** Davis, interview.

137 **IDEA itself would see its growth:** http://www.ideafit.com.

138 **"It was nothing short of incredible":** Davis, interview.

138 **"Getting people physically active":** Video from the 2012 convention.

139 **"Fonda opened everyone's eyes":** Donna Cyrus, interview with the author, New York City, March 2012.

139 **"I realized, okay":** Cyrus, interview.

140 **She spotted the potential:** Cyrus, interview.

140 **"New York set the trend":** Marcello Ehrhardt, interview with the author, Chicago, July 2012.

140 **"Class flies by and you end up drenched":** "Best of New York," *New York Magazine*, March 22, 2004.

141 **"This is your life":** Johnny Goldberg, interview with the author, Montecito, California, November 1, 2011.

141 **"I embarked on that journey":** Goldberg, interview.

142 **"I think it must be like":** Andrea Cagan and Johnny G., *Romancing the Bicycle* (Montecito CA: Johnny G. Publishing, 2000), 14.

143 **in 1994 Mad Dogg athletics:** http://www.maddogg.com.

143 **Among those captivated by Spinning:** Phillip Mills, phone interview with the author, July 2012.

143 **He had captained New Zealand's team:** http://www.lesmills.com.

143 **"handing magazines to people":** Mills, interview.

144 **"The simple reality":** Mills, interview.

144 **"Every bit of research that's ever done":** Mills, interview.

144 **As of 2012 Les Mills:** http://www.lesmills.com.

145 **"getting kind of bored doing fitness shows":** Steinfeld, interview.

146 **Even Bowflex, the hugely successful:** "Nearly 800,000 Bowflex Machines Recalled," NBCNews.com, November 16, 2004.

146 **In 1992 a "cease and desist" order:** Federal Trade Commission ruling *In the matter of Consumer Direct, Inc., et al.*, October 29, 1990.

146 **In its 2002 ruling:** "FTC Charges Three Top-Selling Electronic Abdominal Exercise Belts with Making False Claims," press release, May 8, 2002.

146 **The FTC then set up:** "FTC Charges."

147 **"You got to use the stuff":** Steinfeld, interview.

8. FITNESS TODAY

149 **Atop the list was 24-Hour Fitness:s** Stuart Goldman, "Top 100 Clubs," *Club Industry* (Summer 2012): 26.

149 **Financier Theodore J. Forstmann:** IBISworld Industry report, *Gym, Health, and Fitness Clubs in the U.S.* (July 2012): 25.

149 **Not far behind in revenue:** Goldman, "Top 100 Clubs."

150 **In 2010 Life Time staged:** Steve Stenzel, *Examiner.com*, March 7, 2010.

150 **Bally Total Fitness clocked in at number 5:** Goldman, "Top 100 Clubs."

150 **In New York State alone:** Press release from Office of the New York State Attorney General, "Consumer Complaints Lead to Health Club Sales Reforms," February 2004.

150 **The purchase of Crunch:** Cyrus, interview.

151 **"'I don't have a full gym'":** Caro, interview.

152 **At its 2012 convention:** Documents handed out at the convention and speech by IHRSA president Joe Moore.

153 **"Pieces of equipment that require":** Clawson, interview.

154 **As an industry:** IBISworld Industry report, "Gym and Exercise Equipment Manufacturing in the U.S." (December 2011).

155 **Between 2008 and 2012:** Evelyn M. Rusli, "Investors Put Some Muscle behind Popular Fitness Trend," *New York Times*, March 9, 2012, B5.

155 **A venture capital group:** Rusli, "Investors Put Some Muscle," B5.

156 **"Hey, George Bush became president":** Joe Kita, "The Power of P90X," *Men's Health*, December 18, 2010.

156 **he started flogging P90X:** "BeachBody: Thinking beyond the Infomercial," *Bloomberg Business Week*, November 18, 2010.

156 **"If you look at direct marketing folks":** Kita, "The Power of P90X."

157 **The prototype was Barry's Bootcamp:** Catherine Saint Louis, "Boot Camps Vie to Make You Sweat," *New York Times*, November 10, 2011, E1.

157 **"What separates us":** Saint Louis, "Boot Camps Vie to Make You Sweat," E1.

157 **At IDEA Davis was:** Davis, interview.

157 **At the opposite end:** "Top Ten Health Club Trends for 2012," available at http://ww.ihrsa.org.

158 **Between 1999 and 2011:** IBISworld Industry report, "Personal Trainers in the U.S." (December 2011).

158 **"Once stereotyped as the domain":** Catherine Rampell, "A Jobs Boom Built on Sweat in an Age of Belt-Tightening," *New York Times*, June 30, 2012.

158 **"Most of the people":** Stuart Goldman, "Planet Fitness Ends Personal Training," *Club Industry* (December 9, 2010).

158 **"I actually blame the big-box clubs":** Goldman, "Planet Fitness Ends Personal Training."

159 **DVD sales enjoyed a jump:** IBISWorld *Industry Report: Fitness DVD Production in the US*, February 2012.

159 **Tracy Anderson, who sculpted the bodies:** Rampell, "Jobs Boom."

159 **Anytime Fitness increased revenue:** Goldman, "Top 100 Clubs."

160 **IHRSA pointed out that:** IBISWorld *Industry Report.*

161 **The widespread study of yoga:** William J. Broad, *The Science of Yoga* (New York: Simon and Schuster, 2012).

161 **Its enthusiasts ranged:** Robert Love, *The Great Oom: The Improbable Birth of Yoga in America* (New York: Viking, 2010).

161 **The year that *Asanas* was published:** Love, *Great Oom.*

161 **he went into an "anesthetic trance":** Love, *Great Oom.*

161 **Bernard was an unabashed showman:** Love, *Great Oom.*

162 **In 1961 a hatha yoga teacher:** Mark Singleton, *Yoga Body* (Oxford and New York: Oxford University Press, 2010), 20.

163 **Well over five *billion* dollars a year:** Vanessa Grigoriadis, "Karma Crash," *New York Magazine*, April 15, 2012.

163 **Among the best known are:** Broad, *The Science of Yoga*, xxiii.

163 **In India Gune was the first:** Broad, *The Science of Yoga*, 24.

163 **Using the prevailing benchmark:** Broad, *The Science of Yoga*, 55.

164 **in a study from the University of California:** Broad, *The Science of Yoga*, 60.

164 **"The Davis study and *Yoga Journal* articles":** Broad, *The Science of Yoga*, 64.

164 **"I was an addict":** Deborah Schoeneman, "Yoga Addict's New Mantra: 'Mix It Up,'" *New York Times*, November 24, 2011, E3.

165 **the *Times* excerpt of his detailed chapter:** William J. Broad, "All Bent Out of Shape," *New York Times Magazine*, January 8, 2012.

165 **Merely sitting too long:** Broad, "All Bent Out of Shape."

165 **He followed it a year later:** William J. Broad, "Wounded Warrior Pose," *New York Times*, "Sunday Review," December 22, 2012.

165 **Its antistress utility figured big:** Broad, "All Bent Out of Shape."

165 **"Our culture is so amped up":** Tom Quinn, interview with the author, Chicago, May 2012.

166 **K. V. Iyer, a famous Indian bodybuilder:** Singleton, *Yoga Body*, 122.

166 **Much has been made:** Pearl, *Legends of the Iron Game*, 2:214.

166 **A longtime mentor of Olympic gold medalist:** Pearl, *Legends of the Iron Game*, 2:209–19.

167 **In 2003, age eighty-two:** Pearl, *Legends of the Iron Game*, 2:212.

168 **Swami Muktananda, who had hundreds of ashrams:** William J. Broad, "Yoga and Sex Scandals: No Surprise Here," *New York Times*, February 28, 2012, D6.

168 **Others charged Swami Satchidananda:** Broad, "Yoga and Sex Scandals."

168 **In 2011 a number of women:** Elena Brower quoted in Broad, "Yoga and Sex Scandals."

168 **Broad, the *Times*'s science reporter:** Broad, "Yoga and Sex Scandals," D1.

168 **He had also dabbled in witchy magic:** Grigoriadis, "Karma Crash."

168 **In 1972 an investigation:** http://fitnessliteracyproject.blogspot.com. See also Robert D. McFadden, "Joe Weider, Creator of Bodybuilding Empire, Dies at 93," *New York Times*, March 25, 2013, B9.

169 **The Federal Trade Commission stepped:** "Body Building Firm to Pay $400,000 in Settlement of FTC Vitamin Case," *Los Angeles Times*, August 20, 1985.

169 **Weider agreed to pay a minimum:** "Body Building Firm to Pay."

169 **"Some have argued that the Weiders":** Alan M. Klein, *Little Big Men* (Albany: State University of New York Press, 1993), 99.

169 **In Klein's view:** Klein, *Little Big Men*.

"His bodybuilding magazines": Leo Schuler, "Ten Most Influential Muscleheads," http://www.t-nation.com, December 30, 2011.

170 **Among those teaching the method:** Lawrence Stanley, esq., "Court Overturns Pilates Trademarks," Balanced Body story and opinion of the U.S. district court linked to the website http://www.pilates.com.

170 **Prelitigation dragged on for four years:** Stanley, "Court Overturns Pilates Trademarks."

170 **"The idea that Gallagher owned 'Pilates'":** Stanley, "Court Overturns Pilates Trademarks."

171 **"Since the ruling":** "Joseph H. Pilates," http://www.pilatesstudioofcentralohio.com.

171 **Bikram Choudhury, already in trouble:** Ben McGrath, "Yoga Wars: Steamed," *New Yorker*, February 6, 2012.

172 **She now creates 150 routines:** http://www.jackis.com.

172 **she choreographs new routines:** http://www.jazzercise.com.

172 **"The difference between an older person":** Jane Fonda, *Prime Time* (New York: Random House, Trade Paperbacks, 2012), 87–88.

172 **Mary Bowen, who became a Jungian analyst:** Bowen, interview.

172 **Carola Trier, a professional dancer:** Marguerite Ogle, "The Pilates Elders," About.com, February 16, 2012.

173 **Clara herself, regarded by many:** Bowen, interview.

173 **"People thought stress testing was dangerous":** Cooper, interview.

173 **"My sources tell me that my history":** Unpublished (and unfinished) autobiography of Bonnie Prudden, courtesy of Myotherapy in Tucson AZ.

174 **"The need for supplements":** Joe Weider, e-mail to author, February 16, 2012.

175 **His proudest achievement:** Weider, e-mail to author, February 16, 2012.

176 **"Hey, there's this new sport":** Casey, "World's Healthiest Man."

176 **In subsequent years Wildman completed:** Casey, "World's Healthiest Man."

176 **"Bob was a very loyal friend":** Wilson, e-mail to the author and friends of Delmonteque, November 22, 2011.

177 **"I've changed the environment of exercise":** Johnny G., interview with the author, Montecito, California, November 1, 2011.

177 **He could barely pull himself:** "A Fitness Mogul, Stricken by Illness, Hunts for Genes," *Wall Street Journal*, November 30, 2006.

178 **"I'm a huge believer":** Nieto, interview.

178 **Subsidized by money he had raised** *Club Insider* (December 2011): 6.

178 **"I believe there's a cure":** Quoted in Blythe Bernhard, "From Success to Significance," *Claremont McKenna College Magazine* (Spring 2006).

178 **On *Late Night with David Letterman*:** Numerous websites, including http://washedupcelebrities.blogspot.com.

9. WHY EXERCISE?

181 **More disturbing, a growing number:** Roni Caryn Rabin, "Diabetes on the Rise among Teenagers," *New York Times*, May 21, 2012.

182 **"You can't work alone":** Linda Powell, interview with the author, Chicago, April 2012.

182 **Recent studies found:** Tony Dokoupil, "Tweets, Texts, Email, Posts. Is the Onslaught Making Us Crazy?," *Newsweek*, July 16, 2012, 27.

183 **"Most important, running is fun":** Jim Fixx, *The Complete Book of Running* (New York: Random House, 1977), 10–11.

184 **Citing "a growing body of science":** Gretchen Reynolds, *The First 20 Minutes* (New York: Hudson Street Press, 2012), 102.

185 **A recent study at the Cooper Institute:** "Lifetime Risks for Cardiovascular Disease," *Journal of the American College of Cardiology* 57, no. 15 (2011).

185 **In 1989, however, he turned apostate:** Kolata, *Ultimate Fitness*, 62–63.

185 **"Moderate levels of physical fitness":** Kolata, *Ultimate Fitness*, 62–63.

186 **"A lot of [those] people":** Gina Kolata, "For Some, Exercise May Increase Heart Risk," *New York Times*, May 30, 2012.

186 **"More running is not needed":** Gretchen Reynolds, "Moderation as the Sweet Spot for Exercise," *New York Times*, June 6, 2012.

187 **"Static stretching should be avoided":** Reynolds, *The First 20 Minutes*, 26.

187 **A much larger study:** Reynolds, *The First 20 Minutes*, 27–28.

187 **She was joined in this assessment:** Kolata, *Ultimate Fitness*, 232.

188 **"'I can't tell you'":** Quoted in Reynolds, *20 Minutes or Less*, 138–39.

188 **Another study of collegiate rowers:** Reynolds, *The First 20 Minutes*, 140.

188 **That said, few were prepared:** "For Some, Exercise May Increase Heart Risk," *New York Times*, May 30, 2012.

189 **Describing a two-day work stint:** Kolata, *Ultimate Fitness*, 69.

190 **Men's obsession with "Ab Flab":** Peter Baker, "What's Wrong with Ab Flab?," http://www.menshealthforum.uk, December 1, 2009.

190 **Even that mantra:** Paul Scott, "Everything You Knew about Good Abs May Be Wrong," *New York Times*, February 22, 2007, E8.

190 **"Exercise needs to become":** Cotton, interview.

191 **Phillip Mills did not exaggerate:** Mills, interview.

191 **He detailed those ideas:** Mills, e-mail to the author, July 2012.

191 **"If we tried very hard":** Mills, interview.

191 **"True 'health' clubs will exist":** Phillip Mills, *Globesity* (New York: Random House, 2011).

192 **In a National Cancer Awareness Survey:** PRNewswire, October 18, 2006.

192 **"American Idle Is Killing Us":** PRNewswire, March 1, 2005.

192 **Cotton, for one, is eager:** Cotton, interview. See also http://www.exerciseeismedicine.com.

192 **"How many times a week":** Cotton, interview. See also http://www.exerciseeismedicine.com.

Index

Figure numbers indicate photos, which appear following p. 102.